D1424317

3) Pms
WL 315
CLA

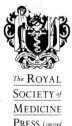

The ROYAL
SOCIETY *of*
MEDICINE
PRESS *Limited*

Parkinson's Disease

SECOND EDITION

in Practice

Carl E Clarke

Reader in Clinical Neurology and Consultant
Neurologist at City Hospital and University
of Birmingham, Birmingham, UK

© 2001, 2007 Royal Society of Medicine Press Ltd
2001 First Edition
2007 Second Edition
Published by the Royal Society of Medicine Press Ltd
1 Wimpole Street, London W1G 0AE, UK
Tel: +44 (0) 20 7290 2921
Fax: +44 (0) 20 7290 2929
Email: publishing@rsm.ac.uk
Website: www.rsmpress.co.uk

Apart from any fair dealing for the purposes of research or private study, criticism or review, as permitted under the UK Copyright Designs and Patents Act, 1988, no part of this publication may be reproduced, stored or transmitted, in any form or by any means, without the prior permission in writing of the publishers or in the case of reprographic reproduction in accordance of the terms of licences issued by the Copyright Licensing Agency in the UK, or in accordance with the terms of licences issued by the appropriate reproduction rights organization outside the UK. Enquiries concerning reproduction outside the terms stated here should be sent to the publishers at the UK address printed on this page.

The rights of Carl Clarke to be identified as author of this work has been asserted by him in accordance with the Copyright, Designs and Patents Act, 1988.

The author is responsible for the scientific content and for the views expressed, which are not necessarily those of the Royal Society of Medicine or of the Royal Society of Medicine Press Ltd.

Although every effort has been made to ensure that, where provided, information concerning drug dosages or product usage has been presented accurately in this publication, the ultimate responsibility rests with the prescribing physician and neither the publisher nor the sponsor can be held responsible for errors or any consequences arising from the use of information contained herein.

British Library Cataloguing in Publication Data
A catalogue record for this book is available from the British Library

ISBN 1-85315-745-7
ISSN 1473-6845

Distribution in Europe and Rest of World:
Marston Book Services Ltd
PO Box 269
Abingdon
Oxon OX14 4YN, UK
Tel: +44 (0) 1235 465 500
Fax: +44 (0) 1235 465 555
Email: direct.order@marston.com

Distribution in Australia and New Zealand:
Elsevier Australia
30–52 Smidmore Street
Marrickville NSW 2204
Australia
Tel: + 61 2 9517 8999
Fax: + 61 2 9517 2249
Email: service@elsevier.com.au

Distribution in the USA and Canada:
Royal Society of Medicine Press Ltd
c/o BookMasters, Inc.
30 Amberwood Parkway
Ashland, OH 44805, USA
Tel: +1 800 247 6553 / +1 800 266 5564
Fax: +1 419 281 6883
E-mail: order@bookmasters.com

Typeset by Phoenix Photosetting, Chatham, Kent, UK
Printed and bound in Spain by Liberdúplex

Dedication

To my wife, Jan, and daughter, Helen, for their love and support
without which this book would never have been written.

About the author

Dr Carl E Clarke BSc MD FRCP is a Reader in Clinical Neurology at the University of Birmingham and Consultant Neurologist at City Hospital, Birmingham, UK. He studied Anatomy and Medicine at the University of Manchester and completed his postgraduate training in Manchester and Yorkshire.

He has been involved in Parkinson's disease research for 20 years. His current interests include systematic reviews of clinical trials in Parkinson's disease and large-scale pragmatic clinical trials such as PD MED, PD SURG and PD OT.

Preface

The first edition of *Parkinson's Disease in Practice* was a great success, not just with general practitioners, but with medical trainees, Parkinson's Disease Nurse Specialists (PDNS), allied health professionals, pharmacists and even patients. This was reflected in it being awarded first prize in the primary care category of the British Medical Association's Medical Book Competition in 2002.

Five years after the first edition was written, the field of Parkinson's disease research has moved on apace. New genetic forms of the condition have given us more insight into the pathophysiology of Parkinson's disease. SPECT scanning is now available to assist in the diagnosis of difficult cases. New medical therapies have come along, such as rasagiline, and new administration routes, such as the rotigotine transdermal patch. Older drugs, such as tolcapone and amantadine, have received a new lease of life. On the horizon, new formulations of older agents offer the promise of continuous dopaminergic stimulation (e.g. modified-release ropinirole and pramipexole). The surgery of Parkinson's disease has also changed radically

since the last version of the book, with the emphasis now being on subthalamic deep-brain stimulation. Recently, the importance of the non-motor complications of the disorder has been realised.

With such a rapid pace of change, a new edition of the book is required to update previous readers and to introduce new readers to the complexity of Parkinson's disease. As in the previous edition, the book reviews the entire spectrum of Parkinson's disease in a concise format with particular emphasis on current therapeutics. Evidence-based medicine rightly remains at the heart of clinical practice in the UK and has been a major interest for the author. The book reflects this, with an evidence-based approach to each therapy area, and a detailed consideration of the very latest guidelines on the diagnosis and management of Parkinson's disease, including those recently published by the National Institute for Health and Clinical Excellence (NICE).

Carl E Clarke
July 2006

Contents

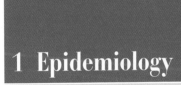

1 Epidemiology

Incidence and prevalence
Mortality

Incidence and prevalence

Incidence is the measure of the number of new cases of a disease occurring over a set period of time for a given location. Incidence rates are not affected by disease survival but are subject to bias according to methods of ascertainment and case definition. The latter point is particularly apposite in Parkinson's disease (PD) because of the difficulties in differential diagnosis (discussed below). The latest review reports the crude incidence rates for PD ranging between 8 and 18/100,000 population/annum. Interestingly, in the stable population of Rochester, Minnesota, US, the incidence of PD varied little between 1945 and 1979 with a range of 16–21/100,000/annum.

> Incidence = number of new cases/year. Incidence of PD is 18/100,000 population; about 10,000 new cases occur in the UK each year

Prevalence is the total number of cases with a condition in a population at a particular point in time. It is affected by survival – prevalence will be closer to incidence in conditions with a short life expectancy, whereas prevalence and incidence will be more disparate in conditions with longer survival (such as PD). Prevalence is also affected by study methodology – estimates from hospital-based surveys produce lower figures than those derived from community-based studies. As a result of these methodological difficulties, prevalence rates in PD vary widely between 18/100,000 (Shanghai,

China) and 328/100,000 (Bombay, India). Less variation is seen if only UK-based studies are examined, which show prevalence rates of 108–164/100,000.

> Prevalence = number of cases in a population at a particular time. There are about 100,000 cases of Parkinson's disease in the UK at any one time

Both incidence and prevalence are markedly affected by the increase in PD with age. The age-specific incidence of PD rises exponentially into the 70s and 80s but then declines in some studies. This decrease is probably an artefact due to poor case ascertainment and the low numbers in these age groups. Age-specific prevalence also increases exponentially over the same age range.

> About 1% of the population over 60 years of age has Parkinson's disease.

PD has been shown in studies to occur more commonly in males than in females. The average male:female ratio based on prevalence studies is 1.35:1, and from incidence studies 1.31:1. These figures are subject to considerable variation, probably due to the underlying age distribution of the populations examined, differences in survival, and access to healthcare.

Crude prevalence studies suggest that the occurrence of PD is more common in Caucasians in Europe and North America, intermediate in Oriental races in Japan and China, and lowest in African races. However, a door-to-door community study in North America showed similar prevalence rates in white and black populations. Thus, ascertainment bias may account for any apparent differences in prevalence between races.

It is impossible to ascertain whether or not there has been any change in the incidence or prevalence of PD over time. However, using the limited data available, adjusted for age and gender, Zhang and Roman have suggested no significant temporal change in either statistic over the past 50 years.

> The ageing population is expected to dramatically increase the number of cases of Parkinson's disease

Mortality

National mortality data

Although national mortality statistics are readily available, they are subject to the following confounding variables:

- accuracy of death certification, with PD often omitted from certificates
- diagnostic difficulties between neurodegenerative conditions mimicking PD – these were compounded in the early part of the past century by cases of post-encephalitic parkinsonism
- changes in the way death certificate data are interpreted centrally
- changing age structure of the population.

Mortality data are most complete for England and Wales. Records date back to 1855, with a break between 1901 and 1920 when PD was not separately classified. The 300% rise in deaths between 1920 and 1989 was mainly due to the ageing population, but was also attributable to increased diagnostic accuracy. This increase continued into the 1990s (Fig. 1.1). Age-specific mortality rates decreased in all age groups below 75 years from 1940 (Fig. 1.2), which was probably due to the dying out of a cohort of patients with post-encephalitic parkinsonism (see later). An increase in age-specific mortality in those over 75 years who presumably had PD was attributed to improved diagnosis.

The dip in mortality in the late 1970s and early 1980s was considered to be due to the introduction of levodopa (chapter 7). This was thought to delay the deaths of predominantly elderly parkinsonian patients for about 5 years, after which there was an increase back to expected levels as this group eventually died and added to the 'expected' deaths.

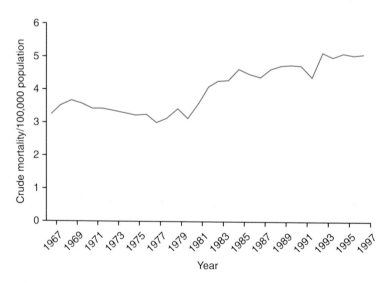

Figure 1.1

Crude mortality rate for PD in England and Wales. Data for 1984–1993 have been corrected for changes in method coding death certificates.

Reproduced with permission from: Clarke CE. Mortality from Parkinson's disease. *J Neurol Neurosurg Psychiatry* 2000; **68**: 254–5.

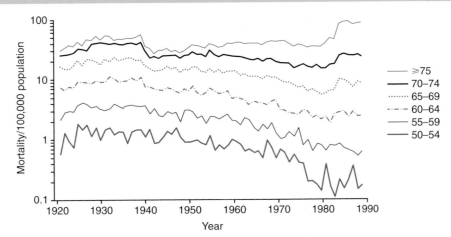

Figure 1.2
Age-specific mortality rates for PD in England and Wales.
Reproduced with permission from: Clarke CE. Mortality from Parkinson's disease in England and Wales 1921–89. *J Neurol Neurosurg Psychiatry* 1993; **56**: 690–3.

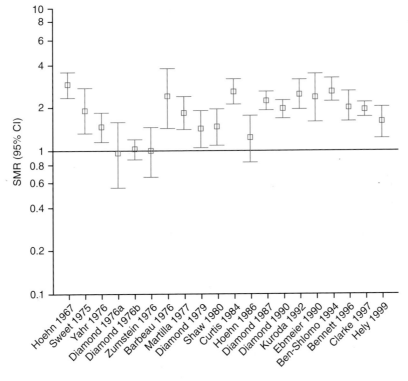

Figure 1.3
Standardised mortality ratios (SMRs) in descriptive and case-control series examining mortality in PD plotted in chronological order of year of publication. Ratios > 1 with 95% confidence intervals that do not overlap one indicate increased mortality in parkinsonian patients.
Reproduced with permission from: Clarke CE. Mortality from Parkinson's disease. *J Neurol Neurosurg Psychiatry* 2000; **68**: 254–5.

Comparable trends in national mortality data have been reported from several Scandinavian countries and the US.

Descriptive and case-control studies

Studies comparing the observed mortality in a group of PD patients with that expected from national mortality statistics are referred to here as descriptive studies. Case-control studies examine mortality rates in two usually matched groups, one with and the other without PD, over the same time period. These study types in PD have been extensively reviewed (Fig. 1.3). They show a fall in the ratio of number of deaths in PD patients to that in controls – the standardised mortality ratio (SMR) – in the early years of levodopa use (late 1970s and early 1980s), but a return to mean SMRs of 1.5–2.0 over the past decade. These studies reported a statistically significant excess mortality rate. In some, the upper 95% confidence interval overlaps the findings of the original Hoehn and Yahr study in the pre-levodopa era.

Thus, although the profound symptomatic impact of levodopa may not be disputed, its effects on mortality were short-lived. Descriptive and case-control studies show that mortality from PD continues to be at levels comparable to those seen before levodopa was introduced. These findings highlight the need for neuroprotective therapy as a matter of urgency.

Since dementia accounts for much of the mortality in PD, more research is required to develop neuroprotective therapies and new treatments for dementia once it has developed.

> Mortality continues to be similar to that in the pre-levodopa era, although levodopa had a short-lived impact on mortality

Further reading

Ben-Shlomo Y. How far are we in understanding the cause of Parkinson's disease? *J Neurol Neurosurg Psychiatry* 1996; **61**: 4–16.

Clarke CE. Does levodopa therapy delay death in Parkinson's disease? A review of the evidence. *Mov Disord* 1995; **10**: 250–6.

Clarke CE. Mortality from Parkinson's disease in England and Wales 1921–89. *J Neurol Neurosurg Psychiatry* 1993; **56**: 690–3.

Clarke CE. Mortality from Parkinson's disease. *J Neurol Neurosurg Psychiatry* 2000; **68**: 254–5.

de Lau LM, Breteler MM. Epidemiology of Parkinson's disease. *Lancet Neurol* 2006; **5**: 525–35.

Hoehn MM, Yahr MD. Parkinsonism: onset, progression, and mortality. *Neurology* 1967; **17**: 427–42.

Schoenberg BS, Anderson DW, Haerer AF. Prevalence of Parkinson's disease in the biracial population of Copiah County, Mississippi. *Neurology* 1985; **35**: 841–5.

Schoenberg BS. Epidemiology of movement disorders. In: Marsden CD, Asbury AK. (eds) *Movement disorders 2.* London: Butterworths, 1987; 17–32.

Tanner CM, Hubble JP, Chan P. Epidemiology and genetics of Parkinson's disease. In: Watts RL, Koller WC. (eds) *Movement disorders: neurologic principles and practice.* New York: McGraw-Hill, 1997; 137–52.

Zhang ZX, Roman GC. Worldwide occurrence of Parkinson's disease: an updated review. *Neuroepidemiology* 1993; **12**: 195–208.

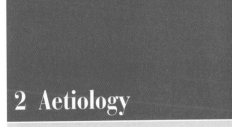

2 Aetiology

Environmental factors
Genetic factors

The cause or causes of Parkinson's disease (PD) remain enigmatic. Time may prove that PD itself is more than one condition, each with more than one cause or perhaps with interacting causative factors. Several potential environmental and genetic factors may be associated with PD.

> There may be several types of idiopathic Parkinson's disease and each may have one or more causes

Environmental factors

Epidemiological studies in this area are comprised of:

- case-control studies, which examine in a group of PD patients and a matched control group the presence or absence of factors that may be causative for the condition. They may deal with present exposures (cross-sectional study) or those in the past (retrospective study)
- prospective cohort studies, in which two groups of people, one exposed to and the other not exposed to a potential cause, are followed over time to assess how many develop PD.

Most PD studies are of case-control design and, therefore, likely to suffer from several potential sources of bias and other problems such as:

- differences in baseline characteristics of the patients and controls (*e.g.* age, sex)
- difficulty in later recall of low exposure to potential toxic agents in both cases and controls ('non-differential misclassification')
- high exposure to an agent may be better recalled by patients with PD ('recall bias')
- multiple significance testing may find associations by chance.

With these caveats in mind, a number of environmental factors have been shown to increase or decrease the risk of PD. These are summarised in Table 2.1 and are briefly discussed below.

MPTP, pesticides and farming

Interest in a potential neurotoxin as a causative factor for PD was re-kindled by the

Table 2.1
Environmental factors associated with PD

	Increased risk	Decreased risk
Toxins	● Pesticides	● Cigarette smoking
	● Rural residence, farming, drinking well-water	● Caffeine (coffee)
	● MPTP*	
	● Manganese, copper	
Infections	● Encephalitis lethargica	
	● Influenza	
Trauma	● Head injury	
Diet	● Vitamin supplements	

*MPTP, 1-methyl-4-phenyl-1,2,3,6-tetrahydropyridine.

discovery that 1-methyl-4-phenyl-1,2,3,6-tetrahydropyridine (MPTP) caused a parkinsonian syndrome similar to PD (Fig. 2.1). This was unwittingly synthesised in the early 1980s by an enterprising chemistry graduate in San Francisco (California, USA), who had been creating his own pethidine (demerol)-analogue for street sale. Intravenous drug abusers who received large doses of MPTP developed a profound parkinsonian syndrome, while about 400 with less exposure and no parkinsonian features are being followed long-term. Three of these patients recently died and autopsy revealed astrocytic and microglial infiltration with extraneuronal melanin in the substantia nigra, suggesting active neuronal loss. This implies that the toxin led to a progressive degenerative process and not a single toxic reaction.

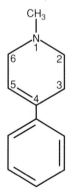

Figure 2.1
Chemical structure of 1-methyl-4-phenyl-1,2,3,6-tetrahydropyridine (MPTP).

MPTP is unlikely to be present in the environment in quantities sufficient to cause PD. It is, however, structurally similar to many other substances, including a number of pesticides. Several case-control studies have shown a small, but significant, increased risk of PD in those exposed to pesticides, rural residence, farming, and drinking well-water. Some of this may be attributable to recall bias. The introduction and increasing use of such agents has only occurred over the past three decades and no corresponding increase in the

incidence of PD has been reported. The population's exposure to such agents is also relatively low, so it has limited significance in terms of public health.

Infections

The outbreak of post-encephalitic parkinsonism following the epidemic of encephalitis lethargica between 1917 and 1926 first raised the possibility that a virus may cause PD. Mortality data for England and Wales suggest that many younger cases of 'PD' in the past who have now died out were in fact due to subclinical encephalitis lethargica. Many other viruses have been proposed, but serological and autopsy support for such theories is lacking.

Head injury

James Parkinson first suggested that head injury may play a part in the genesis of PD. Although several studies have shown an increase in major and minor head injury in PD patients, this is an area where recall bias is particularly likely, so the results must be viewed with caution.

Diet

The potential role of oxidative stress in the pathogenesis of PD has led to the examination of antioxidants, such as vitamins E and C, as neuroprotectants. In some case-control studies, vitamin E has been associated with a low risk of PD, but this has not been found in prospective studies. No relationship between vitamin C intake and PD risk has been found.

Meta-analysis of eight case-control studies and five cohort studies showed a significant decreased PD risk in coffee drinkers (relative risk, 0.69). This may be mediated through the inhibition of the adenosine A_2 receptor by caffeine.

Cigarette smoking

The paradoxical reduced risk of PD in cigarette smokers has been well established for many years from prospective cohort and retrospective case-control series (relative risk – 0.59 for ever-smokers; 0.39 for current smokers). There even appears to be a dose–response relationship. This association is also seen in young-onset PD which excludes the 'competing cause mortality' explanation that smokers liable to PD die from smoking-related disease before they are old enough to manifest the movement disorder. Direct protective effects of smoking have been proposed to explain its beneficial effects but there is no evidence to support such theories. It has also been suggested that a so-called 'parkinsonian personality' trait of introversion and caution may lead presymptomatic individuals to avoid novelty-seeking behaviours such as smoking.

> Cigarette smoking and drinking beverages containing caffeine are protective against Parkinson's disease for reasons that are unknown

Genetic factors

Family studies

Gowers, an English neurologist, drew attention to a familial predisposition to PD over 100 years ago, but it was Mjones in 1949 who published the first large family study based on Swedish cases. Since then, many others have entered the debate with their own series, some concluding that PD is inherited by autosomal dominant inheritance with incomplete penetrance, a few suggesting polygenic inheritance, and others a multifactorial aetiology.

Twin studies

The study of concordance rates in twin pairs offers a unique way to examine the genetic causation of a disease. A higher concordance rate (*i.e.* both twins having the condition) in monozygotic (identical) twins than in dizygotic (non-identical) twins strongly suggests a genetic aetiology. Initial twin studies in PD failed to find a higher concordance rate in monozygotic pairs. However, these studies examined only small numbers, introducing the

possibility of a biased sample, and there remained the possibility that a second twin, unaffected at the time of the study, might have developed the condition in later years. The latter point was addressed in a study using positron emission tomography (PET) which demonstrated lower ^{18}F-fluorodopa uptake and, thus, nigrostriatal neuronal loss in a number of clinically unaffected twins, some of whom have gone on to develop PD, suggesting a higher concordance rate in monozygotic twins.

The latest and largest contribution to this debate has been a study of 19,842 white male US World War II veterans. The concordance rate in 71 monozygotic twin pairs was 0.155 compared with 0.111 in 90 dizygotic pairs (relative risk 1.39; 95% CI 0.63–3.1). This non-significant result should be viewed with caution as it applies only to the male Caucasian population of the US; also, the study only evaluated subjects at one time point, without functional imaging, although they were older than 65 years at the time of screening. Interestingly, all four monozygotic twin pairs with a diagnosis before age 51 years were concordant, compared with only two of the 12 dizygotic twin pairs (relative risk 6.00; 95% CI 1.69–21.3). Although this statistically significant result is in keeping with the finding that large kindreds with autosomal dominant inheritance patterns tend to have a younger age of onset, the small numbers of twin pairs suggests that further work is required for confirmation.

> Monozygotic twins may have a higher concordance rate than dizygotic twins but this needs to be confirmed by further research

Genetic studies

Causative genes

Over the last 10 years, several genes have been found to cause PD. This was made possible by the rapid development of molecular genetic approaches to screening large kindreds with familial PD (Table 2.2).

Table 2.2
Genetic forms of PD

Name	Locus	Gene	Inheritance	Clinical features
Park 1	4q21	α-Synuclein	AD	Young onset; rapid progression
Park 2	6q25.2-27	Parkin	AR	Young onset; slow progression
Park 3	2p13	?	AD	Like PD
Park 4	4p16	?	AD	Like PD
Park 5	4p14	UCHL1	AD	Like PD
Park 6	1p35-36	PINK1	AR	Young onset; slow progression
Park 7	1p36	DJ-1	AR	Young onset
Park 8	12p11.2-13.1	LRRK2/Dardarin	AD	Like PD
Park 9	1p36	?	AR	Parkinsonism; spasticity; dementia; supranuclear palsy
Park 10	1p32	?	?Iceland	Like PD
Park 11	2q36-37	?	?US	?
NR4A2 (NURR1)	2q22-23	Nuclear receptor	AD	Late onset PD

AD, autosomal dominant; AR, autosomal recessive; FTDP, frontotemporal dementia and parkinsonism; UCHL1, ubiquitin carboxy-terminal hydrolase L1; PINK1, phosphatase and tensin homologue deleted on chromosome 10 (PTEN) induced kinase 1; LRRK2, leucine-rich repeat kinase 2.

α-Synuclein (PARK1)

The first gene to be discovered was a single amino acid substitution in the gene for α-synuclein in the large Italian-American Contursi kindred. This dominantly inherited form of parkinsonism was early in onset but was pathologically typical of the idiopathic condition. Although this mutation has been identified in other families, it appears to be a rare cause of familial PD. In nature α-synuclein is a highly conserved protein, being up-regulated in birds during song development. Its function in human neurones is unknown but it readily forms into β-sheets and then aggregates, so the finding of α-synuclein in Lewy bodies, the pathological hallmark of PD (chapter 3), may be a clue to the pathogenetic process.

> The α-synuclein gene mutation is rare in the UK

Parkin (PARK2)

The next gene was discovered in Japanese families with autosomal recessive juvenile-onset disease. The Parkin gene codes for the protein E3 ubiquitin ligase. Ubiquitin is also a component of Lewy bodies but, intriguingly, these patients do not have Lewy bodies at autopsy. In another family, an abnormality in the gene for ubiquitin hydrolase L1 (UCHL1) has been found associated with parkinsonism, although this requires further corroboration.

> The Parkin gene accounts for half of young-onset (< 40 years) autosomal recessive cases in the UK

LRRK2 (PARK8)

Mutations in the LRRK2 gene have been shown to cause a condition very similar to sporadic PD in large families with autosomal dominant PD. Many groups have now screened smaller families with PD and found that LRRK2 mutations occur in around 5%. More recently, it has been shown that LRRK2 mutations account for 0.4–1.6% of cases of sporadic PD with no family history of the condition. The large protein coded for by LRRK2 is likely to be a protein kinase, but how this may take part in the pathogenesis of the condition is unknown.

> LRRK2 mutations account for around 0.4–1.6% of cases of sporadic PD

DJ-1 (PARK7)

Autosomal recessive DJ-1 mutations cause around 1% of cases of young-onset PD. Of particular interest, DJ-1 translocates to the outer mitochondrial membrane which may give a clue to its pathogenetic mechanism.

PINK1 (PARK6)

Similar to Parkin and DJ-1 mutations, mutations in the PINK1 gene cause autosomal recessive young-onset PD. Like DJ-1, the function of PINK1 is linked to mitochondria.

Clinical implications for causative genes

Patients with a clear familial predisposition to PD are rare. Deciding on possible genetic causes in such families can be aided by the useful algorithm given in Healy et al. (2004).

These genetic mutations are relative rare (< 5%) in sporadic cases of PD in which there is no family history of the condition. However, their value in sporadic PD lies more in elucidating possible pathogenetic pathways. So, α-synuclein, Parkin and UCHL1 mutations are involved with the ubiquitination of a synuclein by the cell's waste disposal system, the proteasome. How this leads to neuronal dysfunction and death is unknown. In contrast, PINK1 and DJ-1 may lead to mitochondrial dysfunction (see below).

> Although genetic cases of PD are rare, they may shed light on the pathogenetic pathways of the condition

Susceptibility genes

Sporadic PD is more likely to be caused by the interaction of genetic and environmental factors. To identify these relatively weak candidate genes requires large association studies in which the frequency of the mutation in the PD cases is compared with that in a non-affected control group. Many genes have been studied over the years, mostly those concerned with dopamine metabolism (e.g. MAOB, COMT), but none have been conclusively shown to be implicated in the pathogenesis of PD. More association studies need to be performed and the availability of large banks of DNA from patients with PD will help this search in the future (e.g. PD GEN).

Mitochondrial inheritance

A deficiency of mitochondrial complex 1 has been found in PD, so it is conceivable that the condition may be transmitted through a mitochondrial gene defect. Since mitochondria are inherited through the maternal line, a maternal transmission pattern would thus be expected if this was the case. Although this has not been found in practice, this form of inheritance remains a possibility since most archetypal mitochondrial disorders, such as chronic progressive external ophthalmoplegia and the Kearns-Sayre syndrome, present as sporadic cases. It was recently found that the mitochondrial complex 1 deficiency in humans could be transmitted through isolated mitochondrial deoxyribonucleic acid (DNA) to so-called rho⁰ cells deficient in mitochondria. In the future, the hunt for a mitochondrial gene abnormality is likely to focus on sequencing the mitochondrial genome in patients with low complex 1 activity and a transmissible defect.

Further reading

Ben-Shlomo Y. Smoking and neurodegenerative diseases. *Lancet* 1993; **342**: 1239.

Ben-Shlomo Y. The epidemiology of Parkinson's disease. In: Quinn NP. (ed) *Parkinsonism*. London: Baillière-Tindall, 1997; 55–68.

Burn DJ, Mark MH, Playford ED et al. Parkinson's disease in twins studied with ¹⁸F-dopa and positron emission tomography. *Neurology* 1992; **42**: 1894–900.

de Lau LM, Breteler MM. Epidemiology of Parkinson's disease. *Lancet Neurol* 2006; **5**: 525–35.

Gu M, Cooper JM, Taanman JW, Schapira AHV. Mitochondrial DNA transmission of the mitochondrial defect in Parkinson's disease. *Ann Neurol* 1998; **44**: 177–86.

Healy DG, Abou-Sleiman PM, Wood NW. PINK, PANK, or PARK? A clinicians' guide to familial parkinsonism. *Lancet Neurol* 2004; **3**: 652–62.

Langston JW, Ballard PA, Tetrud JW, Irwin I. Chronic parkinsonism in humans due to a product of meperidine-analog synthesis. *Science* 1983; **219**: 979–80.

Langston JW, Forno LS, Tetrud J et al. Evidence for active nerve cell degeneration in the substantia nigra of humans years after 1-methyl-4-phenyl-1,2,3,6-tetrahydropyridine exposure. *Ann Neurol* 1999; **46**: 598–605.

Marsden CD. Twins and Parkinson's disease. *J Neurol Neurosurg Psychiatry* 1987; **50**: 105–6.

Nicholl DJ, Bennett P, Hiller L et al. A study of five candidate genes in Parkinson's disease and related neurodegenerative disorders. European Study Group on Atypical Parkinsonism. *Neurology* 1999; **53**: 1382–3.

Parkinson J. *An essay on the shaking palsy*. London: Sherwood, Neely, and Jones, 1817.

Piccini P, Burn DJ, Ceravolo R et al. The role of inheritance in sporadic Parkinson's disease: evidence from a longitudinal study of dopaminergic function in twins. *Ann Neurol* 1999; **45**: 577–82.

Riggs JE. Cigarette smoking and Parkinson's disease: the illusion of a neuroprotective effect. *Clin Neuropharmacol* 1992; **15**: 88–99.

Tanner CM, Hubble JP, Chan P. Epidemiology and genetics of Parkinson's disease. In: Watts RL, Koller WC. (eds) *Movement disorders: neurologic principles and practice*. New York: McGraw-Hill, 1997; 137–52.

Tanner CM, Ottman R, Goldman SM et al. Parkinson's disease in twins: an etiologic study. *JAMA* 1999; **281**: 341–6.

Ward CD, Duvoisin RC, Ince SE et al. Parkinson's disease in 65 pairs of twins and in a set of quadruplets. *Neurology* 1983; **33**: 815–24.

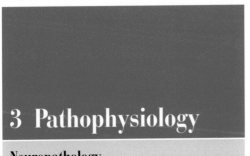

3 Pathophysiology

Neuropathology
Neurochemistry
Basal ganglia functional anatomy

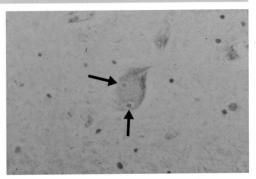

Figure 3.1
Nigral dopaminergic cell containing typical Lewy bodies (arrows).

Neuropathology

There are three pathological hallmarks of Parkinson's disease (PD):

- Lewy bodies
- neuronal death in the pars compacta of the substantia nigra
- the removal of neuromelanin from dead cells by microglia.

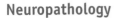

Lewy bodies

Lewy bodies are eosinophilic intraneuronal inclusions named after a German pathologist. They are found in the catecholaminergic nuclei affected in PD, along with the cerebral cortex, thalamus, brainstem, intermediolateral column of the spinal cord, sympathetic ganglia, and myenteric plexus of the gastrointestinal tract. The classical nigral Lewy body (Fig. 3.1) is composed of three layers:

- densely staining central core
- larger outer body
- surrounding halo.

In the cortex, the layers within the Lewy body are less distinct, but in the hypothalamus and sympathetic ganglia they may be multiple, may overlap and may even merge into elongated inclusions. Electron microscopy of a typical Lewy body reveals a sunflower appearance comprised of a body and a halo, which are composed of neurofilaments and a core made of

granular material. The immunocytochemical staining characteristics of the granular material are complex but include phosphorylated neurofilaments, tubulin, microtubulin-associated protein (MAP) and ubiquitin. Ubiquitin is a highly conserved 76 amino acid protein that normally conjugates with other proteins to label them for non-lysosomal adenosine triphosphatase (ATPase)-dependent proteolysis in an intracellular organelle called the proteosome. Anti-ubiquitin staining is particularly useful in identifying the rarer cortical Lewy body.

Although much information has been accumulated on the Lewy body, its precise role in the pathophysiology of PD remains unknown.

The prevalence of incidental Lewy bodies at autopsy in patients without signs of PD steadily rises from 4% in the seventh decade to 33% in the 11th decade. It is well established that clinical signs of PD do not develop until normal striatal dopamine levels are reduced by 80% and cell loss in the substantia nigra reaches 50%. This clearly suggests a presymptomatic phase of the illness and that those with incidental Lewy bodies at postmortem might have developed the condition had they lived. This evidence, coupled with the exponential rise in the prevalence of PD with age (chapter 1), raises important public health issues as the populations of developed nations age significantly over the next few decades.

About 4% of asymptomatic people in their seventh decade and 33% in their 11th decade will have Lewy bodies, suggesting that they have presymptomatic Parkinson's disease

Neuronal death in the substantia nigra and Lewy bodies are the pathological hallmark of Parkinson's disease

Although the Lewy body is an essential feature in PD, it can also be seen in other conditions including Alzheimer's disease, pantothenate kinase associated neurodegeneration (PKAN; Hallervorden-Spatz disease), multiple system atrophy (MSA; see chapter 4), progressive supranuclear palsy (PSP; see chapter 4), and the Parkinsonian-dementia complex of Guam. Presumably, it is a common end-product of neuronal degeneration.

Neuronal death and neuromelanin removal

The loss of dopaminergic neurones from the substantia nigra pars compacta is an essential feature of PD. However, other catecholaminergic nuclei also suffer cell loss, including the ventral tegmental area, locus coeruleus, hypothalamus, raphé nuclei and sympathetic ganglia. The resulting loss of neuromelanin from the substantia nigra leads to the depigmentation of this structure at postmortem (Fig. 3.2). The role of neuromelanin in the genesis of PD is unknown.

Braak staging

Recently, Braak and colleagues have used a synuclein immunostaining techniques to document the stereotyped progression of Lewy bodies from brainstem and olfactory nuclei, through the substantia nigra pars compacta, to the cortex (Table 3.1). This work supports the possibility of presymptomatic PD in those with a restricted number of Lewy bodies in brainstem structures. However, this pathological model does have problems which include its inability to explain the presentation of Lewy body dementia with cognitive dysfunction appearing before any motor features.

Neurochemistry

Neurotransmitter depletion

The profound depletion of dopamine from the major output projection of the substantia nigra, the corpus striatum (caudate and putamen), was first reported by Ehringer and Hornykiewicz in 1960. This ultimately formed the rationale for the therapeutic breakthrough with the introduction of levodopa replacement therapy. Further work demonstrated similar dopamine

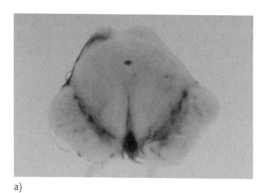
a)

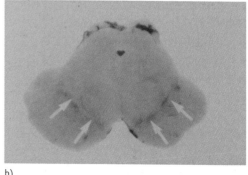
b)

Figure 3:2
Midbrain section from: (a) control and (b) a patient with PD (arrows indicate depigmentation).

Table 3.1
Braak pathological staging in PD

Braak stage	Nuclei involved
Stage 1	Dorsal motor nucleus of vagus and intermediate reticular zone
Stage 2	Stage 1 plus caudal raphe and gigantocellular reticular nuclei and locus coeruleus–subcoeruleus complex
Stage 3	Stage 2 plus midbrain lesions, particularly pars compacta of substantia nigra
Stage 4	Stage 3 plus cortex in temporal mesocortex and allocortex (CA2-plexus). Not neocortex
Stage 5	Stage 4 plus high order sensory association areas of neocortex and prefrontal neocortex
Stage 6	Stage 5 plus first order sensory association areas of neocortex and premotor areas and occasionally primary sensory and motor areas

depletion in the mesocorticolimbic and hypothalamic systems. The loss of 80% striatal dopamine before clinical features of PD develop suggests that good compensatory mechanisms exist. These consist of:

- a presynaptic increase in the turnover of dopamine in surviving neurones
- the postsynaptic increase in dopamine receptor sensitivity.

> About 80% of dopamine must be lost from the striatum before parkinsonian symptoms develop – the brain, therefore, has excellent compensatory mechanisms

The loss of neurones from the locus coeruleus in the brainstem leads to a depletion of cortical noradrenaline. Similarly, 5-hydroxytryptamine (5-HT) is reduced in the striatum due to raphé nucleus involvement.

Non-catecholaminergic neurones are also affected in PD. Loss of cholinergic neurones from the nucleus basalis of Meynert leads to reduced cholinergic innervation of the neocortex and hippocampus. Reductions in the peptides substance P, met-enkephalin, cholecystokinin and somatostatin in the basal ganglia in PD have been demonstrated, but the functional consequences of these changes are not known.

Oxidative stress and free radicals

Oxidative stress occurs when there is excess production of free radicals. Free radicals are a series of molecules and chemical species that contain one or more unpaired electrons (Table 3.2). Electrons are usually paired and have opposite spins. With unpaired electrons, free radicals become highly reactive and oxidise agents by extracting electrons from other substances. This may result in damage to deoxyribonucleic acid (DNA), enzymes, other cellular proteins and unsaturated fatty acids. Natural defence mechanisms exist to destroy free radicals – enzymes such as superoxide dismutase (SOD) and glutathione peroxidase, and chemicals such as vitamin E, ascorbate, glutathione, urea compounds and ubiquinone can all scavenge and destroy free radicals.

A number of abnormalities in PD support the possibility that oxidative stress may play a part in the pathogenetic process. Glutathione levels in the nigra are reduced and some studies have shown reduced glutathione peroxidase activity. SOD levels are increased in both the cytosol and mitochondria in PD nigral neurones, suggesting increased exposure to superoxide radicals. Polyunsaturated fatty acids, malondialdehyde and hydroperoxides (products

Table 3.2
Examples of free radical species

Superoxide anion (O_2^{-})
Hydroxyl radical ($HO^{\bullet}$)
Nitric oxide (NO)
Peroxynitrite ($ONOO^{-}$)
Triplet oxygen ($^{3}O_2$)
Singlet oxygen ($^{1}O_2$)

of lipid membrane damage) are increased in PD nigra. In addition, 8-hydroxydeoxyguanosine, a product of DNA damage, is increased in PD substantia nigra.

Iron can catalyse oxidative reactions that produce free radicals. Increased iron levels have been found in the substantia nigra in PD and may contribute to neuronal damage by increasing oxidative stress. A deficiency of 35% in respiratory chain complex I activity in mitochondria in PD may also predispose patients to oxidative stress.

> Oxidative stress, increased iron and deficient mitochondrial complex I may be implicated in the pathogenesis of Parkinson's disease

Thus, multiple, tantalising, pathological, neurochemical and biochemical abnormalities have been reported to occur in PD. At present, it is not known which of these is primary and which secondary, or even artefactual. Future work on abnormal gene products may allow a synthesis of these various abnormalities in familial cases of the disorder, which in turn is likely to help our understanding of sporadic cases (Fig. 3.3).

Basal ganglia functional anatomy

Considerable strides have been made over the past 20 years in understanding the functional anatomy of the basal ganglia. The combination of neuroanatomical tracing studies, 2-deoxy-D-glucose autoradiography and microelectrode recordings have allowed a 'wiring diagram' of the basal ganglia to be assembled (Fig. 3.4). As with any 'simple' explanation for a complex set of cerebral functions, this model has been found lacking in more recent years, but it still provides a detailed insight into certain aspects of PD physiology and has allowed a rational approach to novel surgical techniques in PD.

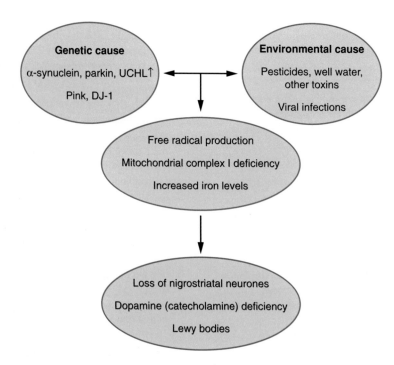

Figure 3.3
Postulated pathophysiology of PD.

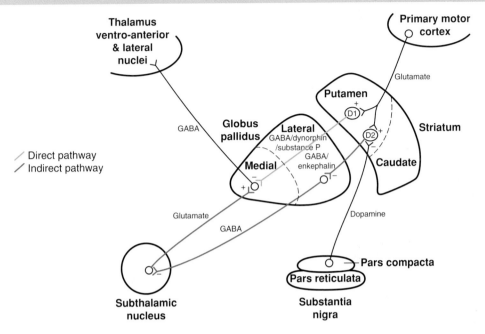

Figure 3.4
Major connections of the basal ganglia.
+ = excitatory neurotransmitter; – = inhibitory neurotransmitter.

The pathway through the basal ganglia passes from the premotor cortex through the striatum and globus pallidus to the thalamus, and then back to the supplementary motor cortex. Activity in this loop is modulated by the substantia nigra which acts like a motor car accelerator, and the subthalamic nucleus (STN) which acts like a brake. In PD, the substantia nigra is defective and thus the accelerator fails to work and the patient slows down. Following a stroke involving the STN, the brake is lost and the patient develops contralateral involuntary movements (hemiballismus/ hemichorea syndrome).

In normal conditions, the substantia nigra acts like a car accelerator on the basal ganglia, and the subthalamic nucleus like a brake. Damage to the substantia nigra in Parkinson's disease slows the patient down, while damage to the subthalamic nucleus speeds the patient up

On a more complex level, the functions of the nigra and STN are mediated through two pathways (Fig. 3.4):

- **direct pathway** – this is comprised of gabaminergic neurones in the striatum projecting to the medial segment of the globus pallidus; these, in turn, inhibit gabaminergic neurones passing to the ventroanterior and ventroposterior nuclei of the thalamus. The inputs to this pathway are a glutamatergic projection from the premotor cortex and the nigral dopaminergic pathway

- **indirect pathway** – this is comprised of gabaminergic neurones in the striatum projecting to the lateral segment of the globus pallidus, which inhibit the gabaminergic neurones to the STN; these, in turn, inhibit the glutamatergic projection to the medial segment of the globus pallidum, which stimulates the gabaminergic neurones passing to the ventroanterior and ventroposterior nuclei of thalamus.

In PD, dopamine deficiency results in increased activity in striatopallidal gabaminergic fibres (Fig. 3.5). This inhibits the lateral pallidal gabaminergic neurones to the STN. The glutamatergic STN projection to the pallidum is thereby stimulated which increases the firing of medial pallidal gabaminergic neurones to the thalamus. Interestingly, these changes are the opposite to what happens in experimental models of chorea and ballism.

In levodopa-induced dyskinesia in PD, the opposite changes would be expected but this is not quite what is found. Instead of metabolic activity in the medial pallidum decreasing to normal with levodopa treatment, it increases. This could only be due to increased activity in the direct pathway from the striatum to the medial pallidal segment since the STN was inhibited. This leads to excessive inhibition of

medial pallidal firing, as is seen in experimental models of chorea.

The above must be an oversimplification, since the peptides co-localised with GABA play no part in the model. Also, the somatotopic point-to-point projection of neurones is not taken into account, nor is the fact that each single line in the diagram represents around 10,000 individual neurones. However, it does explain why lesioning the STN (i.e. subthalamic nucleotomy) or switching off the STN (i.e. STN stimulation) in PD leads to improvement as the overactive subthalamopallidal glutamatergic pathway is disrupted. This is also the reasoning behind the search for glutamate antagonists for use in PD.

> Overactivity in the glutamate pathway between the STN and medial segment of the globus pallidus in Parkinson's disease is central to new therapeutic strategies (i.e. subthalamic nucleus lesions and stimulation)

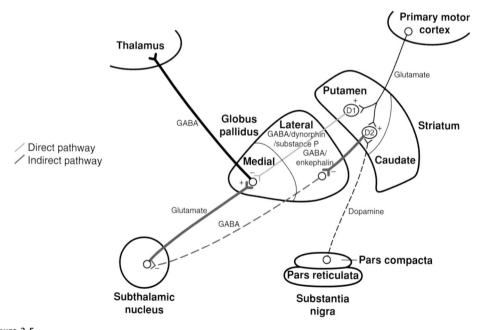

Figure 3.5

Changes in the basal ganglia in PD.

Dotted lines represent decreased activity in pathway; solid lines represent increased activity in pathway; + = excitatory neurotransmitter; − = inhibitory neurotransmitter.

Further reading

Alexander GE, DeLong MR. Microstimulation of the primate neostriatum: II. Somatotopic organization of striatal microexcitable zones and their relation to neuronal response properties. *J Neurophysiol* 1985; **53**: 1433–46.

Braak H, Tredici K, Rüb U, de Vos RA, Jansen Steur EN, Braak E. Staging of brain pathology related to sporadic Parkinson's disease. *Neurobiol Aging* 2003; **24**: 197–211.

Crossman AR. Primate models of dyskinesia: the experimental approach to the study of basal ganglia-related involuntary movement disorders. *Neurosci* 1987; **21**: 1–40.

Ehringer H, Hornykiewicz O. Verteilung von noradrenalin und dopamin (3-hydroxytyramin) im gehirn des menschen und ihr verhalten bei erkrankungen des extrapyramidalen systems. *Klin Wochenschr* 1960; **38**: 1236–9.

Fearnley J, Lees AJ. Parkinson's disease: Neuropathology. In: Watts RL, Koller WC. (eds) *Movement disorders: neurologic principles and practice*. New York: McGraw-Hill, 1997; 263–78.

Fearnley JM, Lees AJ. Ageing and Parkinson's disease: substantia nigra regional selectivity. *Brain* 1991; **114**: 2283–301.

Flaherty AW, Grabiel AM. Anatomy of the basal ganglia. In: Marsden CD, Fahn S. (eds) *Movement disorders 3*. New York: Butterworth-Heinemann, 1994; 3–27.

Forno LS. Pathology of Parkinson's disease. In: Marsden CD, Fahn S. (eds) *Movement disorders*. London: Butterworths, 1982; 25–40.

Jellinger K. The pathology of parkinsonism. In: Marsden CD, Fahn S. (eds) *Movement disorders 2*. London: Butterworths, 1987; 124–65.

Mitchell IJ, Clarke CE, Boyce S et al. Neural mechanisms underlying parkinsonian symptoms based upon regional uptake of 2-deoxyglucose in monkeys exposed to 1-methyl-4-phenyl-1,2,3,6-tetrahydropyridine. *Neurosci* 1989; **32**: 213–26.

Mizuno Y, Ikebe SI, Hattori N et al. Aetiology of Parkinson's disease. In: Watts RL, Koller WC. (eds) *Movement disorders: neurologic principles and practice*. New York: McGraw-Hill, 1997; 161–82.

Schapira AHV. Pathogenesis of Parkinson's disease. In: Quinn NP. (ed) *Parkinsonism*. London: Baillière-Tindall, 1997; 15–36.

4 Clinical features

Diagnostic signs and symptoms
Other features
Treatment-related complications
Differential diagnosis
Clinical rating scales

Diagnostic signs and symptoms

The cardinal diagnostic signs in early
Parkinson's disease (PD) are:

- hypokinesia and bradykinesia
- rigidity
- rest tremor.

Hypokinesia and bradykinesia

Hypokinesia refers to the poverty of movement
in PD. Patients lose facial expression and arm
swing when walking. By contrast, bradykinesia
refers to slowness of movement. The term
akinesia implies no movement at all but, as
this rarely occurs in PD, the former two more
precise terms are preferred, although they are
often imprecisely combined as bradykinesia.
The difficulties generated by hypokinesia and
bradykinesia cause the patient most difficulty
with motor function.

Rigidity

The patient experiences this as stiffness
affecting all muscle groups, both axial and
limb. On examination, rigidity is appreciated as
a resistance to passive movement. When
looking for rigidity, the clinician must always
remember to re-inforce the movement by asking
the patient to move the contralateral limb
(Froment's sign). Thus, as the examined wrist is

flexed and extended, the patient should flex
and extend the contralateral arm at the
shoulder. That said, the pathophysiological
basis of both rigidity and the effects of re-
inforcement are not fully understood.

Extrapyramidal rigidity differs from spasticity.
Resistance to passive movement remains
constant through the range of motion in
extrapyramidal rigidity, while in spasticity there
is a velocity-dependent increase in tone
followed by relaxation which is called the
clasp-knife phenomenon as it resembles the
closure of a penknife.

Rigidity may feel smooth, so-called 'lead-pipe',
or jerky due to superimposed tremor when it is
referred to as 'cogwheeling'.

Rest tremor

Tremor is an involuntary rhythmical alternating
movement. In PD, it is initially seen in one
upper limb with intermittent opposition of the
thumb and index finger, which is called 'pill
rolling' as though the patient is rolling a pill
between the thumb and index feature. The
frequency is typically 4–6 Hz. This spreads to
the ipsilateral leg and then the other limbs as
the condition progresses. Tremor is the first
symptom of PD in about 75% of patients, but
up to 20% of cases never develop tremor at any
stage of the illness.

> Tremor is the first symptom of Parkinson's disease
> in ~75% of patients

It is important to differentiate clearly between
parkinsonian tremor and essential tremor (ET)
which is discussed later. Parkinsonian tremor
occurs at rest while ET occurs when maintaining
a posture (postural tremor) and performing an
action (action tremor). Parkinsonian tremor is
also clearly different from a cerebellar intention
tremor, in which the amplitude of the tremor
increases towards the point of intent. Inability
to get the patient's limb at rest to observe a
parkinsonian rest tremor is a common problem
and is often best seen with the patient walking

with both arms by his or her side. It has been known for many years that a postural tremor can be seen in PD in association with a rest tremor; however, it was recently found that this is often delayed in onset ('re-emergent'), unlike ET in which it begins as soon as the posture is adopted, and that it is of the same frequency as the rest tremor.

Precision of diagnosis

A study in north Wales has shown the diagnostic error rate of parkinsonian syndromes in the community to be 50%.

Studies from several brain banks in the early 1990s demonstrated that precision of the clinical diagnosis of PD was particularly poor. The UK Parkinson's Disease Society Brain Research Centre study of 100 consecutive patients with a clinical diagnosis of PD showed that only 76 had Lewy bodies in the brain at autopsy. Pedantic application of the previously reported diagnostic criteria (Table 4.1) only reduced this error from 24% to 18%. The diagnostic error rate in large trials where the diagnosis of PD was made by an expert was only 6–8%. Since an accurate diagnosis has fundamental implications in terms of treatment response and prognosis, it is suggested that all patients with suspected PD are referred to a specialist with experience in diagnosing and treating the condition.

Postural instability

Postural instability is a fundamental feature of PD but, as it develops later in the course of the condition, cannot be used as an early diagnostic feature. It is usually associated with a stooped posture with flexion of the cervical and thoracic spine. Imbalance is manifest as a tendency to fall either forwards or backwards. The slow shuffling gait at this stage of the condition combined with the postural difficulties leads to the forward 'festinating' gait. Patients can also lose balance and shuffle backwards culminating in a fall ('retropulsion').

Posture can be examined at the bedside by standing the patient with his or her feet

Table 4.1
UK Parkinson's Disease Society Brain Bank Diagnostic Criteria for PD

STEP 1 Diagnosis of parkinsonian syndrome
Bradykinesia (slowness of initiation of voluntary movement with progressive reduction in speed and amplitude of repetitive actions) and at least one of the following:

- muscular rigidity
- 4–6 Hz rest tremor
- postural instability not caused by primary visual, vestibular, cerebellar or proprioceptive dysfunction

STEP 2 Exclusion criteria for PD
- History of repeated strokes with stepwise progression of parkinsonian features
- History of repeated head injury
- History of definite encephalitis
- Oculogyric crises
- Neuroleptic treatment at onset of symptoms
- > 1 affected relative
- Sustained remission
- Strictly unilateral features after 3 years
- Supranuclear gaze palsy
- Cerebellar signs
- Early severe autonomic involvement
- Early severe dementia with disturbances of memory, language and praxis
- Babinski's sign
- Presence of a cerebral tumour or communicating hydrocephalus on computed tomography scan
- Negative response to large doses of levodopa (if malabsorption excluded)
- MPTP* exposure

STEP 3 Supportive prospective positive criteria for PD: three or more required for diagnosis of definite PD
- Unilateral onset
- Rest tremor present
- Progressive disorder
- Persistent asymmetry affecting the side of onset most
- Excellent (70–100%) response to levodopa
- Severe levodopa-induced chorea
- Levodopa response for ≥ 5 years
- Clinical course of ≥ 10 years

*MPTP, 1-methyl-4-phenyl-1,2,3,6-tetrahydropyridine (Fig. 2.1).

slightly apart and then sharply pulling the patient backward (the 'pull test').

Falls represent a dangerous feature in later disease with the likelihood of fractures. If falls emerge very early in the course of a parkinsonian syndrome, progressive supranuclear palsy (PSP, see later) is the more likely diagnosis.

> Hypokinesia and bradykinesia, rigidity and rest tremor are the diagnostic features of Parkinson's disease

Other features

Motor freezing

Freezing is the inability to initiate movement ('gait ignition failure') or the sudden stopping of movement when encountering an external stimulus such as a doorway. The neural mechanism of this intriguing symptom is unknown but it creates major difficulties for patients and does not respond to dopaminergic medication. Freezing should be differentiated from the sudden 'switching off' (immobile phase) that patients with levodopa-induced motor complications develop (chapter 7).

Paradoxical kinesia is the brief return of near normal mobility in PD in response to an urgent external stimulus such as an alarm bell.

Speech disorder

The speech disorder of PD is complex (page 85). The voice becomes monotonous and low in volume (hypophonia), with poor rhythm that can lead to repetition of the first syllable (palilalia).

Dysphagia

Dysphagia is seen later in the disease (page 86). It has been shown to respond to levodopa.

Dystonia

Dystonia of the hand or foot can be seen in early untreated PD, but more commonly after levodopa therapy (chapter 7). Thus, writer's cramp can develop before other features of the disease. Calf cramp with or without obvious dystonic plantar flexion and inversion of the ankle is common after treatment for some years. Involuntary extension of the great toe ('striatal toe') can also be seen and, occasionally, flexion of the fingers into the palm.

Frozen shoulder

Relative immobility and rigidity can lead to a frozen shoulder.

Cardiovascular

Postural hypotension

Postural hypotension of a mild degree can be seen in later PD and can be exacerbated by levodopa and dopamine agonists.

Oedema

Relative immobility and rigidity can produce postural lower limb oedema but this can be caused by dopamine agonists.

Autonomic detrusor hyper-reflexia

Mild autonomic dysfunction is common in later PD, although this should be differentiated from the earlier and more profound autonomic problems seen in multiple system atrophy (MSA). Detrusor hyper-reflexia leads to urinary frequency and urgency with, more rarely, incontinence in later PD.

Constipation

Constipation is almost universal in PD from the early stages of the illness.

Excessive salivation

This is common in late PD but does not respond to antiparkinsonian therapy. Often, the best advice for patients is to chew sugar-free chewing gum which forces them to swallow.

Sleep disorders

Sleep disorders are common in PD (page 74). Some are due to other pathologies in this elderly population, such as prostatism. Others, such as vivid dreams and nightmares, are likely to be due to medication such as selegiline (chapter 6). Inability to turn over in bed is extremely common and is due to the deliberate use of short-acting medication, such as levodopa, during the day and not at night. Leg dystonia often occurs while the patient is in the 'off phase' in bed.

The restless legs syndrome (RLS) is common in PD and can precede the condition by some years. It is comprised of irresistible leg movements, often accompanied by creeping sensations in the legs. The movements are worse with rest, particularly when trying to sleep. Effective treatment relies on levodopa or the dopamine agonists, suggesting that this condition is in some way related to dopaminergic deficiency.

Sleep behaviour disorder (RBD) is also associated with PD. Normally, during rapid eye movement (REM) sleep, we are atonic despite dreaming. In RBD, however, patients act out vivid dreams, sometimes in a violent fashion. Although RBD is not specific to PD, it can be the harbinger of the condition. Clonazepam 0.25–1.00 mg at night can reduce the symptoms of RBD but can give rise to excessive sedation or drowsiness.

Mental health

Dementia

The cumulative prevalence of dementia in PD is 80% (chapter 10). Typically, this gives rise to:

- impaired executive function
- fluctuating confusion
- visual hallucinations.

These problems become worse as a result of dopaminergic medication and can be precipitated by withdrawing the patient from the familiar environment of his or her home to respite care or hospital.

Dementia in PD can be difficult to differentiate from the more common Alzheimer's disease and multiple cerebral infarct dementia as all three

can display parkinsonian signs. The value of an expert opinion from a clinician experienced in this diagnostic dilemma is inestimable. Some patients present with dementia and no motor signs of PD, so-called 'dementia with Lewy bodies' (DLB).

Depression

Depression is present in about 40% of patients with PD at any one time and is often overlooked (chapter 10). A recent quality-of-life study showed that it accounted for 40% of the reduction in quality of life in PD compared with the 17% reduction caused by disease severity and medication.

Treatment-related complications

Although levodopa has a major beneficial effect in PD, it rapidly became clear after its introduction that it causes significant motor adverse events in long-term therapy. These are considered in detail in chapter 7.

Differential diagnosis

In view of the high diagnostic error rate in non-experts, all patients with suspected PD should be referred to a local expert clinician and their PD service.

Essential tremor

The most common diagnostic error is believing that every patient with an isolated tremor has PD; statistically, the majority of such patients will have ET. Recent work has suggested that ET is an autosomal dominant condition, the penetrance of which depends on age; thus, most affected individuals will have developed it by the time they have reached their 60s, if they live that long.

ET is a very common condition. Although prevalence studies in this area suffer from poor case-ascertainment, the prevalence of ET is likely to be in the region of 1500/100,000 population (compared with PD at about 150/100,000). A general practitioner will, therefore, see about 10 times as many cases of ET as PD.

> Essential tremor is 10 times more common than Parkinson's disease, and it is often misdiagnosed as Parkinson's disease in general practice

Patients with ET most commonly present with a history of tremor of the upper limbs for a number of years, often more than five years. This contrasts with PD in which the tremor has usually been present for less than 2 years. The tremor occurs when maintaining a posture (*i.e.* holding the arms outstretched) and when performing an action (*i.e.* holding a tea-cup or screwdriver). The tremor of PD is mainly a rest tremor which disappears with posture and action. ET can affect the head, leading to titubation, and, rarely, the voice. It can be disabling in some cases, which is the reason for recently dropping the epithet 'benign' from the title.

> Essential tremor usually comprises an upper limb postural tremor and an action tremor, lasting more than 2 years, whereas Parkinson's disease has a rest tremor presenting for less than 2 years

Treatment is confined to β-blockers (*e.g.* propranolol) and anti-epilectic drugs (*e.g.* primidone, topiramate) if tolerated, although functional neurosurgery can be useful for more severe patients.

> ET may affect the head and voice

Presentation of a parkinsonian syndrome

For patients presenting with a parkinsonian syndrome of hypokinesia/bradykinesia and rigidity, with or without tremor, the differential diagnosis is much larger (Table 4.2).

In practice, the rarest of these conditions can rapidly be dismissed after taking the patient's history and performing an examination using a checklist of 'red flags' (Table 4.3).

Table 4.2
Differential diagnosis of a parkinsonian syndrome

- PD
- Drug-induced parkinsonism (*e.g.* phenothiazines)
- Multiple cerebral infarct state
- Trauma – pugulistic encephalopathy
- Toxin-induced parkinsonism (*e.g.* MPTP, carbon monoxide, manganese, copper)
- Parkinson's plus syndromes
  - Progressive supranuclear palsy (PSP)
  - Multiple system atrophy (MSA)
    - Shy Drager syndrome
    - Olivopontocerebellar atrophy
    - Striatonigra degeneration

Table 4.3
Clinical features suggesting a parkinsonian syndrome is not due to PD

- History of severe cerebral trauma, stroke, exposure to neurotoxins or anti-dopaminergic agents
- Absence of rest tremor
- Symmetrical signs
- Associated ophthalmoplegia, pyramidal or cerebellar signs
- Associated autonomic dysfunction
- Rapid disease progression
- Poor response to levodopa

A group of Parkinson's plus syndromes initially appears so similar to PD that differentiation can be extremely difficult, even in experienced hands. Of these, progressive supranuclear palsy (PSP) and multiple system atrophy (MSA) are the two most common.

Progressive supranuclear palsy

PSP, or Steele-Richardson-Olszewski syndrome, typically presents with a symmetrical parkinsonian syndrome associated with early postural instability and falls, with the later development of a supranuclear ophthalmoplegia in which vertical, then horizontal eye movements are lost. Patients can develop:

- upper motor neurone signs in the limbs
- a pseudobulbar palsy with dysphagia and dysarthria

- upper motor neurone signs of slow spastic tongue movements
- a brisk jaw jerk.

> Dementia is common in later stages of progressive supranuclear palsy

Preterminally, patients often suffer from a dementia. Rarer features can be useful in diagnosis, *e.g.* cervical dystonia leading to retrocollis (*i.e.* neck extension) and levator disinhibition which is a form of blepharospasm. The condition progresses more rapidly than PD and the parkinsonism is poorly responsive to levodopa. Pathologically, the condition is typified by the finding of neurofibrillary tangles and atrophy in the cerebral cortex, striatum, substantia nigra and brainstem. The tangles contain abnormally phosphorylated tau protein, which is a microtubular-associated protein involved in the axonal transport of vesicles.

> Progressive supranuclear palsy progresses faster than Parkinson's disease and does not respond as well to levodopa

Differentiating PSP from PD can be difficult as specific signs, mainly the eye movement disorder, are frequently absent within the first few years of diagnosis. The early postural instability and falls should lead to the suspicion of PSP. A patient with a parkinsonian syndrome who has falls in the first 2 or 3 years of developing the condition is likely to have PSP. Patients with PD tend to fall much later in course of the condition, after around 8–10 years.

> There is an early history of falls in progressive supranuclear palsy, and later supranuclear ophthalmoplegia with loss of downward and upward gaze and then horizontal eye movements

Multiple system atrophy

MSA is a relatively new term for a group of conditions that were previously thought to be unique. Recently, the similar terminal clinical features of these conditions and the discovery of a common glial cytoplasmic inclusion body have led to their unification under this specific heading.

Patients with MSA present in three broad categories, which loosely reflect the old nomenclature:

- Shy-Drager syndrome – present with autonomic dysfunction such as erectile failure, impotence, urinary incontinence and retention, faecal incontinence, postural hypotension and syncope
- olivopontocerebellar atrophy – present with cerebellar signs such as gait and limb ataxia and incoordination
- striatonigral degeneration – present with a relatively pure parkinsonian syndrome.

As the condition progresses, considerable overlap occurs in the clinical features and others such as upper motor neurone signs develop.

> Multiple system atrophy presents with autonomic disturbance, cerebellar syndrome or parkinsonian syndrome, with an overlap in clinical features as the disease progresses

As with PSP, some rare but specific signs can be useful in diagnosis. These include:

- laryngeal dystonia leading to stridor and sleep apnoea, for which elective tracheostomy can be life-saving
- disproportionate antecollis, *i.e.* neck flexion with less kyphosis than is seen in PD
- stimulus-sensitive myoclonus, which is best elicited by a pin prick of the outstretched pronated hand.

The response to levodopa is poor in most patients but some can improve, especially with large doses, and a few may even develop dyskinesia, especially oro-facial. It is important to note that dementia never develops in MSA and is an exclusion criterion for the diagnosis.

Disease progression is more rapid than in PD but slower than in PSP.

> Dementia does not develop in multiple system atrophy. Progression of multiple system atrophy is faster than in Parkinson's disease and the response to levodopa is poor

As with PSP, differentiation of MSA from PD can be difficult in the initial stages when specific features are absent. Rapid progression and poor response to large doses of levodopa (about 1000 mg levodopa with a decarboxylase inhibitor, *e.g.* Sinemet Plus 10 tablets daily) should alert the clinician to the possibility of MSA, especially in younger patients (with the mean age of onset being 54 years in MSA). Early autonomic features, such as impotence and urinary problems, strongly suggest MSA.

Specific features of MSA include laryngeal dystonia (stridor and sleep apnoea), disproportionate antecollis and stimulus-sensitive myoclonus

Drug-induced parkinsonism

Parkinsonism can be induced by various drugs. For example, patients given prochlorperazine to treat non-specific dizziness may develop a parkinsonian syndrome as a result of its anti-dopaminergic activity. The parkinsonism settles when such agents are withdrawn, but this can take months. Some patients may even require dopaminergic therapy.

Multiple cerebral infarct state

A multiple cerebral infarct state leading to 'arteriosclerotic pseudo-parkinsonism' is a common diagnostic problem, particularly in the secondary care setting. However, most of these patients present with a classical *marché à petits pas* gait (*i.e.* shuffling with small steps) with few, if any, signs of parkinsonism in the upper limbs. This is referred to as 'lower-half parkinsonism'. Such patients generally do not respond to levodopa and progress rapidly, usually developing other features of a multiple

infarct state such as dementia, incontinence, transient ischaemic attacks and stroke. The only treatment is to attend to cerebrovascular risk factors such as hypertension, smoking, diabetes, *etc.* Computed tomography brain scanning may be necessary to exclude hydrocephalus in some cases.

Wilson's disease

This is an autosomal recessive condition with accumulation of copper within the liver leading to cirrhosis, and within the striatum leading to tremor, parkinsonism, chorea, and/or dystonia usually with some psychiatric features such as depression and personality change. It is, therefore, crucial in all young (< 50-year-old) patients with parkinsonism to have serum caeruloplasmin and urine copper studies to exclude this disease.

Differential diagnosis, referral and treatment

Due to the considerable problems in accurately diagnosing the cause of a parkinsonian syndrome, even in expert hands, it is generally accepted that it is preferable for patients with suspected PD to be referred to a secondary care physician with a special interest in such movement disorders, before a firm diagnosis is made. This is supported by NICE guidelines.

> Treatment for Parkinson's disease should not be initiated in the primary care setting without specialist advice

It is also best that such patients are referred before treatment is commenced because:

- they may not need treatment if they do not have PD
- treatment may mask the diagnosis of PD
- they may not have significant functional disability from their PD
- they may best be treated with dopamine agonist monotherapy if they are relatively young with PD.

Primary care physicians should refer patients with suspected parkinsonism to a neurologist or geriatrician with an interest in Parkinson's disease for the most accurate diagnosis and the most appropriate treatment

Clinical rating scales

Clinical rating scales are used to measure the severity of PD in clinical trials. Whilst detailed consideration of these scales is beyond the scope of this book, some knowledge of them is useful to understand the trials presented in later sections (Tables 4.4 and 4.5).

Table 4.4
Hoehn and Yahr staging scale

Stage of PD	Severity of PD
Stage 1.0	Unilateral involvement only
Stage 1.5	Unilateral and axial involvement
Stage 2.0	Bilateral involvement without impairment of balance
Stage 2.5	Mild bilateral involvement with recovery on retropulsion (pull) test
Stage 3.0	Mild-to-moderate bilateral involvement, some postural instability but physically independent
Stage 4.0	Severe disability, still able to walk and to stand unassisted
Stage 5.0	Wheelchair bound or bedridden unless aided

Table 4.5
Common outcome measures used in clinical trials in PD

Scale	Type of measure	Number of items (score range)
Motor and ADL scales		
Unified Parkinson's Disease Rating Scale (UPDRS)*	Mentation (part I) – impairment	4 (0–16)
	Activities of daily living (part II) – disability	13 (0–52)
	Motor (part III) – impairment	27 (0–108)
	Complications of treatment (part IV) – impairment	11 (0–23)
	Total UPDRS score (total of parts I to IV above) – mixed	(0–199)
Patient on/off diary cards	Impairment	–30 or 60 min epochs
Quality-of-life scales		
Parkinson's Disease Questionnaire (PDQ) 39	Mixed impairment and disability	39
EuroQol EQ5	Mixed impairment and disability	5 and graticule
Short Form 36 (12)	Mixed impairment and disability	36 (12)

The UPDRS is currently being updated; higher scores indicate worse function.

Further reading

Cummings JL. Depression and Parkinson's disease: a review. *Am J Psychiatry* 1992; **4**: 443–54.

Findley L, Peto V, Pugner K et al. The impact of Parkinson's disease on quality of life: results of a research survey in the UK. *Mov Disord* 2000; **15 (Suppl 3)**: 179.

Gibb WRG, Lees AJ. The relevance of the Lewy body to the pathogenesis of idiopathic Parkinson's disease. *J Neurol Neurosurg Psychiatry* 1988; **51**: 745–52.

Golbe LI. Progressive supranuclear palsy. In: Watts RL, Koller WC. (eds) *Movement disorders: neurologic principles and practice*. New York: McGraw-Hill, 1997; 279–95.

Hoehn MM, Yahr MD. Parkinsonism: onset, progression, and mortality. *Neurology* 1967; **17**: 427–42.

Hughes AJ, Daniel SE, Kilford L, Lees AJ. Accuracy of clinical diagnosis of idiopathic Parkinson's disease: a clinico-pathological study of 100 cases. *J Neurol Neurosurg Psychiatry* 1992; **55**: 181–4.

Jankovic J, Schwartz KS, Ondo W. Re-emergent tremor of Parkinson's disease. *J Neurol Neurosurg Psychiatry* 1999; **67**: 646–50.

Koller WC, Busenbark KL. Essential tremor. In: Watts RL, Koller WC. (eds) *Movement disorders: neurologic principles and practice*. New York: McGraw-Hill, 1997; 365–85.

Lees AJ. The Steele-Richardson-Olszewski syndrome (progressive supranuclear palsy). In: Marsden CD, Fahn S. (eds) *Movement disorders 2*. London: Butterworth, 1987; 272–87.

Lennox GG, Lowe JS. Dementia with Lewy bodies. In: Quinn NP. (ed) *Parkinsonism*. London: Baillière-Tindall, 1997; 147–66.

Litvan I. Progressive supranuclear palsy and corticobasal degeneration. In: Quinn NP. (ed) *Parkinsonism*. London: Baillière-Tindall, 1997; 167–85.

Quinn N. Multiple system atrophy – the nature of the beast. *J Neurol Neurosurg Psychiatry* 1989; **Suppl**: 78–89.

Quinn N. Multiple system atrophy. In: Marsden CD, Fahn S. (eds) *Movement disorders 3*. Oxford: Butterworth-Heinemann, 1994; 262–81.

Schenck CH, Bundlie SR, Mahowald MW. Delayed emergence of a parkinsonian disorder in 38% of 29 older men initially diagnosed with idiopathic rapid eye movement sleep behaviour disorder. *Neurology* 1996; **46**: 388–93.

Wenning GK, Quinn NP. Multiple system atrophy. In: Quinn NP. (ed) *Parkinsonism*. London: Baillière-Tindall, 1997; 187–204.

5 Investigations

Functional imaging
Structural imaging
Neurochemical techniques
Neurophysiological techniques
Other investigations
Combinations of investigations

The diagnosis of Parkinson's disease (PD) is made on clinical grounds in the majority of patients. In recent years, considerable effort has gone into developing diagnostic tests for the condition. This has been productive with the recent licensing of Ioflupane (^{123}I-FP-CIT; DaTSCAN®) single photon emission computed tomography (SPECT) which is helpful in making the diagnosis in a small number of patients. Many more tests have been evaluated, but at present these require further work before they become established.

> The diagnosis of Parkinson's disease relies on clinical judgement in the majority of cases and is best made by a clinician with considerable experience in the condition.

Assessing the value of a putative diagnostic test for PD requires a number of standard properties to be evaluated:

- Sensitivity – number with condition and positive test (true positives) divided by number with the condition
- Specificity – number without condition with negative test (true negatives) divided by number without the condition

- The 'best' tests have both high sensitivity and specificity (approaching 1.0)
- The best way to judge the balance between sensitivity and specificity is with receiver–operator characteristics (ROC) curves which guide the choice of test result 'cut-off'.

Functional imaging

Single photon emission computed tomography (SPECT)

In positron emission tomography (PET), a positron-emitting radioactive isotope is tagged to a molecule of interest or tracer which is then administered to the patient, usually by intravenous injection. This is taken up by the area of interest. The isotope then emits positrons which annihilate with electrons producing two high-energy γ-rays at 180° to one another. Co-incidental hits by the γ-rays at two opposing sodium iodide detectors can be registered allowing measurement of absolute tissue concentration of the isotope and thus the molecule of interest (Fig. 5.1). This can be processed to produce traditional two-dimensional images (i.e. tomographs) and, more recently, three-dimensional parametric maps of tracer uptake.

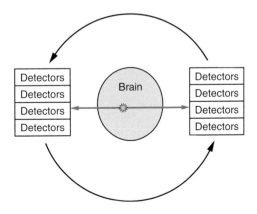

Figure 5.1
Principle of PET. Green arrows represent release of two γ-rays at 180° to each other.

In single photon emission computed tomography (SPECT), isotopes which release only one γ-ray are used, such as ^{123}Iodine and ^{99m}Technetium. These isotopes are easier to produce and use since they have longer half-lives. Consequently, different tracers are used in SPECT (Table 5.1). The result is a more practical and less expensive tool than PET, but at the expense of spatial resolution. The labelled cocaine derivatives ^{123}I-FP-CIT and ^{123}I-β-CIT have most commonly been used with SPECT to label the presynaptic dopamine re-uptake site and, thus, the presynaptic neurone.

The isotopes are still quite short-lived. ^{123}I-FP-CIT (DaTSCAN®) has been available in the UK for several years, with the isotope produced in The Netherlands and transported by rail or air overnight for the nuclear medicine departments who require it for scans the next day. Because of the larger distances involved, ^{123}I-FP-CIT is still not available in the US. Ligands using longer-lived isotopes, such as ^{99m}Technetium, are being developed to address this need.

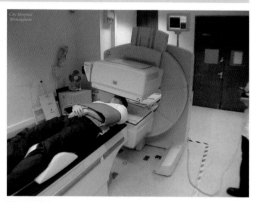

Figure 5.2
Gamma camera used in SPECT.
Courtesy of Dr A Notgi.

is not difficult. The recent NICE guidelines stated that ^{123}I-FP-CIT SPECT should be available to experts with experience in the differential diagnosis of PD.

There is a lot of evidence to support the use of ^{123}I-FP-CIT SPECT in people with postural and/or action tremor of the upper limbs to differentiate essential tremor from a dopamine deficiency state (*i.e.* PD, PSP, MSA, *etc.*). The scan is normal in essential tremor and normal people, with the striatum looking like inverted 'commas' (Fig. 5.3a). There is an asymmetric loss of uptake in the putamen in PD which, in early disease, looks like a loss of the tail of the normal striatal 'comma' (Fig. 5.3b). In late PD, uptake in both putamen is lost leaving the uptake in the two caudate nuclei looking like 'full stops' (Fig. 5.3c).

---

^{123}I-FP-CIT SPECT can be used in patients with upper limb tremor to differentiate essential tremor from parkinsonism.

Table 5.1
SPECT radioligands and their binding sites

Biological application	Radioligand
Dopamine transporter	^{123}I-FP-CIT (^{123}I-N-ω-fluoropropyl-2β-carboxymethoxy-3β-(4-iodophenyl)nortropane)
	^{123}I-β-CIT (123I-N-[2-fluoroethyl]-2β-carbomethoxy-3β-(4-iodophenyl)tropane)
	^{99m}Tc-TRODAT
	^{99m}Tc-technepine

^{123}I-FP-CIT imaging can be performed with a standard gamma camera which is commonly available in most district general hospitals (Fig. 5.2). The interpretation of the images is quite straight forward in most cases. So, setting up a new service to deliver this imaging

It is not useful in separating PD from parkinsonism due to multiple cerebral infarcts as ^{123}I-FP-CIT SPECT can be abnormal in both conditions. Recent work has demonstrated the value of this technique in differentiating parkinsonism due to neuroleptic medication and psychogenic parkinsonism from a dopaminergic deficiency state.

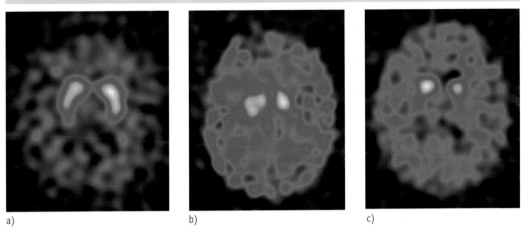

a)   b)   c)

Figure 5.3
^{123}I-FP-CIT SPECT scans. (A) Essential tremor with normal uptake. (B) Early Parkinson's disease with asymmetric loss of uptake in the putamen seen as loss of the tail of the 'comma'. (C) Late Parkinson's disease with severe loss of putamen uptake bilaterally seen as loss of both tails resulting in two 'full stops'.
Courtesy of Dr A Notgi.

> ^{123}I-FP-CIT SPECT can be used to differentiate parkinsonism due to neuroleptic medication and psychogenic parkinsonism (normal scan) from a dopaminergic deficiency state (abnormal scan)

Several clinical trials using SPECT or PET to follow the progression of PD found that 4–14% of people with a clinical diagnosis of PD had normal imaging at the start of the trial. Further long-term clinical follow-up of these people is on-going, but it seems likely that these cases were misdiagnosed rather than representing false negatives.

The uptake of ^{123}I-FP-CIT can be reduced by cocaine, amphetamines, methylphenidate, bupropion, sertraline, and benztropine which should be stopped for around 1 week before imaging.

Positron emission tomography (PET)

Table 5.2 shows the tracers used in PET and their applications. The drawback of this technique is its expense because of the need to manufacture the isotopes immediately before injection using an expensive cyclotron. As a result, there are few PET scanners available,

although the number in the UK has just increased for its application in cancer detection.

The most valuable PET tracer in PD work has proved to be ^{18}F-6-fluorodopa (^{18}F-dopa). This is taken up by the nigrostriatal dopaminergic neurones and converted into ^{18}F-dopamine and then its metabolites. The rate of accumulation of ^{18}F is dependent on the transport of ^{18}F-dopa into the brain, the neurones and then the vesicles versus its rate of breakdown.

^{18}F-dopa PET was first examined in PD in the early 1980s. Uptake was reduced by around 30% at the onset of the disease. This compares with the 80% or greater loss of dopamine and dopaminergic neurones which highlights the compensatory mechanisms available in the striatum. In twin studies, ^{18}F-dopa PET identified preclinical PD in apparently unaffected co-twins.

Fascinating follow-up ^{18}F-dopa PET studies in PD have shown an annual decline in uptake of around 9–12%. Extrapolating backwards, this suggests a preclinical period of 3–6 years which is in keeping with data on the rate of nigral cell loss. This provides a window for neuroprotective

Table 5.2
PET radioligands and their binding sites

Biological application	Radioligand
Blood flow	$H_2{}^{15}O$, ^{99m}Tc-HMPAO, ^{133}Xe
Oxygen metabolism	$^{15}O_2$
Glucose metabolism	^{18}F-2-fluoro-2-deoxyglucose (^{18}FDG)
Dopamine storage	^{18}F-6-fluorodopa (^{18}F-dopa)
Dopamine transporter	^{11}C-dihydrotetrabenazine (DHTBZ)
Dopamine re-uptake sites	^{11}C-CFT, ^{11}C-RTI-32, ^{11}C-RTI-121
	^{11}C-nomifensine
	^{123}I-β-CIT, ^{123}I-FP-CIT, ^{123}I-IPT
Dopamine D_1 sites	^{11}C-SCH 23390
Dopamine $D_{2/3}$ sites	^{11}C-raclopride
	^{11}C-methylspiperone (MSP)
	^{18}F-fluoroethylspiperone
	^{76}Br-bromospiperone (BSP)
	^{123}I-iodobenzamide (IBZM)
	^{123}I-epidipride
MAOB activity	^{11}C-deprenyl
Opioid binding	^{11}C-diprenorphine

therapies if only we can identify potential patients at this preclinical stage. Much debate surrounds the use of ^{18}F-dopa PET and ^{123}I-FP-CIT uptake as an outcome measure in neuroprotection trials in PD (see chapter 6).

Recently, work examining glucose metabolism with ^{18}F-fluorodeoxyglucose (^{18}F-FDG) PET has suggested that this technique may be able to differentiate accurately between controls, PD patients and those with MSA or PSP. Further confirmation of this is necessary.

The poor availability of PET means that it is unlikely to become widely available for the differential diagnosis of PD.

Cardiac MIBG scintigraphy

In PD, there is a loss of the postganglionic sympathetic innervation of the heart due to the loss of noradrenergic neurones. This is not seen in the other parkinsonian syndrome which commonly gives rise to autonomic failure, multiple system atrophy (MSA). These postganglionic noradrenergic nerves can be labelled with ^{123}I-meta-iodobenzylguanidine (^{123}I-MIBG). Some groups have proposed that cardiac ^{123}I-MIBG can be used to differentiate

the autonomic failure of PD from MSA, but the sensitivity and specificity of this technique in the early stages of these conditions remains to be proven.

Magnetic resonance spectroscopy

Proton magnetic resonance spectroscopy (MRS) can provide information on the concentrations of intermediary metabolites in a small volume of cerebral tissue. The metabolite of largest concentration is N-acetylaspartate (NAA) which is found principally in neurones and their processes. The creatine (Cr) peak is taken as a marker of energy status and that for choline (Cho) as an indicator of membrane synthesis and degradation. Additional smaller peaks can be seen at short echo times representing glutamate, aspartate and inositol. Review of MRS studies in parkinsonian syndromes demonstrates considerable heterogeneity in the results which preclude any firm conclusions being reached at present. Further, large, multicentre trials are required preferably using absolute quantitation of tissue metabolite concentrations.

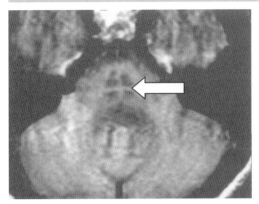

Figure 5.4
Proton density MRI in MSA showing increased signal in the brain stem (so-called 'hot-cross bun' sign, arrow). Reproduced from Watts RL, Koller WC. *Movement Disorders. Neurological Principles and Practice*. New York: McGraw-Hill, 1997; 301.

Structural imaging
Computed tomography

The comparatively poor spatial resolution of computed tomography (CT) limits its value in the differential diagnosis of parkinsonian syndromes, although it can demonstrate brainstem and cerebellar atrophy in MSA. Its main use is in excluding other pathology in clinically atypical cases, such as multiple cerebral infarct state, but the requirement for scanning should be the prerogative of the secondary care physician with expertise in these conditions.

Magnetic resonance imaging

The superior resolution of magnetic resonance imaging (MRI) provides for more precise estimates of brain stem and cerebellar atrophy in MSA and software developments now allow volumetric analysis of such structures. However, MRI has also demonstrated signal changes in some patients with MSA and PSP (Fig. 5.4).

Various combinations of atrophy and signal changes have been examined for their discriminatory value in the differential diagnosis of established parkinsonian syndromes. The conclusion from this work is

that an abnormal MRI is highly specific to MSA or PSP, whereas a normal MRI does not exclude the diagnosis because of the low sensitivity of the investigation. This low sensitivity hampers the value of MRI as a diagnostic test, but it has the advantage of being readily available.

Neurochemical techniques
Acute apomorphine and levodopa challenge tests

The striking clinical response to oral levodopa and the subcutaneously administered dopamine agonist apomorphine in PD raised the possibility that acute challenges with these substances may be useful diagnostic tests for the condition.

A systematic review of the small studies examining this issue located nine trials. These evaluated one group with a clinical diagnosis of PD for some time (*n* = 306), along with a separate group who were felt to have PD plus conditions such as MSA and PSP (*n* = 130). Acute challenge tests with either levodopa, apomorphine or both were performed and the responses monitored by a number of clinical tests using thresholds to define PD or non-PD. This was then compared with the diagnostic 'gold standard', the response to chronic levodopa therapy given over several months in the clinic. Aside from significant methodological problems related to the defining of threshold levels, both acute challenge tests showed similar sensitivity and specificity in the diagnosis of PD as chronic levodopa therapy (Fig. 5.5). Also, the heterogeneity tests in the meta-analyses and logistic regression analysis failed to show statistically significant variation between studies in the sensitivities or specificities. Since no significant difference was found between the acute tests and chronic levodopa therapy, there is no advantage gained by using the acute challenge tests since patients are going on to have chronic levodopa therapy. Most will receive levodopa, or a dopamine agonist, so the value of the acute tests is minimal.

a)

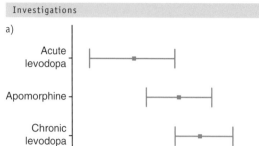

b)

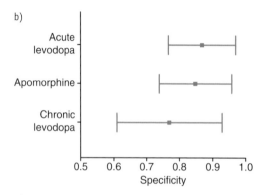

Figure 5.5
Meta-analysis of the (a) sensitivity and (b) specificity of acute challenge tests with apomorphine and levodopa compared with chronic levodopa therapy in the differentiation of PD from other Parkinson's plus conditions. Bars represent mean and 95% confidence intervals.
Reproduced with permission from Clarke CE, Davies P. Systematic review of acute levodopa and apomorphine challenge tests in the diagnosis of idiopathic Parkinson's disease. *J Neurol Neurosurg Psychiatry* 2000; **69**: 590–4.

> Acute challenge tests with levodopa and apomorphine are of no additional diagnostic value to chronic therapy with levodopa and probably dopamine agonists

The real challenge for these diagnostic tests is in very early PD when diagnostic uncertainty is at its height. Systematic review of the four studies examining acute challenge tests in newly diagnosed untreated PD patients (*n* = 209) also showed that these tests show no advantage over chronic levodopa therapy (Fig. 5.6).

Although acute apomorphine challenges may not be of any value in the diagnosis of PD, this does not preclude their use later in the disease to either demonstrate a continued response to dopaminergic therapy or as a prelude to apomorphine therapy.

Clonidine growth hormone stimulation test

The α-2-adrenoreceptor agonist clonidine increases growth hormone (GH) secretion in healthy controls after intravenous injection by an action at the hypothalamic level. Reports that GH levels in response to clonidine increased in untreated patients with PD, but not MSA, raised the possibility that this test may be useful in differentiating the conditions. However, more recent work has failed to replicate this work, possibly due to the considerable variability in growth hormone levels. In the future, other more reliable tests of hypothalamic function may prove to be of value in this situation.

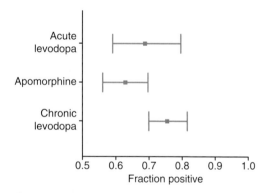

Figure 5.6
Meta-analysis of apomorphine, acute levodopa, and chronic levodopa challenge tests in patients with newly diagnosed IPD. Bars represent mean and 95% confidence intervals.
Reproduced with permission from Clarke CE, Davies P. Systematic review of acute levodopa and apomorphine challenge tests in the diagnosis of idiopathic Parkinson's disease. *J Neurol Neurosurg Psychiatry* 2000; **69**: 590–4.

Neurophysiological techniques

Anal sphincter electromyography

A small group of anterior horn cells in the sacral spinal cord termed Onuf's nucleus degenerate in MSA but not PD. This leads to denervation of the external urethral and anal sphincters and, thus, causes the symptoms of bladder and bowel disturbance seen in MSA. The use of electromyography (EMG) of the urethral sphincter as a diagnostic test for MSA yielded a sensitivity of 0.62 and specificity of 0.92. Subsequent work using urethral sphincter EMG and/or the better tolerated anal sphincter EMG, using different cut-off criteria, yielded similar results (0.74 and 0.89 sensitivity for MSA, respectively). However, denervation of the external anal sphincter has also been seen in five of 12 patients with PSP (sensitivity 0.42).

Much more work is required on this technique, in particular, diagnostic thresholds using receiver–operator characteristics (ROC) curves. Its application is also limited by it being an unpleasant procedure for the patient.

Other investigations

Smell testing

Around 80% of people with PD have an impaired sense of smell (hyposomia), particularly for oregano (pizza aroma). Since olfaction can be objectively tested with a battery of different odours, it has been evaluated in the differential diagnosis of PD.

Objective smell testing has a moderate sensitivity (76–91%) and specificity (78–88%) in differentiating people with PD from controls, but there are few data on its ability to differentiate PD from other parkinsonian syndromes. Odour recognition is also diminished in other neurodegenerative conditions, such as Alzheimer's disease.

In view of the simplicity of this kind of test, further research should be done in this area.

Combinations of investigations

Much more organised investment is required to complete the evaluation of existing tests for PD and to develop new ones. Many investigations are expensive with limited availability, so it would be particularly useful to develop inexpensive tests based on serum or cerebrospinal fluid biomarkers or more sophisticated bedside tests, such as olfaction, eye movements, neuropsychological testing and detailed movement analysis.

Combining two or more tests may improve diagnostic accuracy. This is particularly applicable to less expensive investigations. Also, head-to-head comparisons of promising diagnostic tests should be undertaken, *e.g.* ^{123}I-FP-CIT SPECT with objective smell identification.

Once neuroprotective therapies for PD have been developed, it will be crucial to diagnose the condition early, perhaps even before it becomes symptomatic. This will require inexpensive, sensitive, specific, and safe tests which can be used to screen large numbers of the population.

Further reading

Booij J, Tissingh G, Winogrodzka A, van Royen EA. Imaging of the dopaminergic neurotransmission system using single photon emission tomography in patients with parkinsonism. *Eur J Nuclear Med* 1999; **26**: 171–82.

Brooks DJ. PET and SPECT studies in Parkinson's disease. In: Quinn NP. (ed) *Parkinsonism*. London: Baillière Tindall, 1997; 69–87.

Burn DJ, Mark MH, Playford ED *et al.* Parkinson's disease in twins studied with ^{18}F-dopa and positron emission tomography. *Neurology* 1992; **42**: 1894–900.

Burn DJ, Sawle GV, Brooks DJ. Differential diagnosis of Parkinson's disease, multiple system atrophy, and Steele-Richardson-Olszewski syndrome: discriminant analysis of striatal ^{18}F-dopa PET. *J Neurol Neurosurg Psychiatry* 1994; **57**: 278–84.

Clarke CE, Ray PS, Speller JM. Failure of the clonidine growth hormone stimulation test to differentiate multiple system atrophy from advanced idiopathic Parkinson's disease. *Lancet* 1999; **353**: 1329–30.

Clarke CE, Davies P. Systematic review of acute levodopa and apomorphine challenge tests in the diagnosis of idiopathic Parkinson's disease. *J Neurol Neurosurg Psychiatry* 2000; **69**: 590–4.

Eardley I, Quinn NP, Fowler CJ et al. The value of urethral sphincter electromyography in the differential diagnosis of parkinsonism. Br J Urol 1989; **64**: 360–2.

Fearnley JM, Lees AJ. Aging and Parkinson's disease: substantia nigra regional selectivity. Brain 1991; **114**: 2283–301.

Kimber JR, Watson L, Mathias CJ. Distinction of idiopathic Parkinson's disease from multiple-system atrophy by stimulation of growth-hormone release with clonidine. Lancet 1997; **349**: 1877–81.

Kraft E, Schwarz J, Trenkwalder C, Vogl T, Pfluger T, Oertel WH. The combination of hypointense and hyperintense signal changes in T2-weighted magnetic resonance imaging sequences. A specific marker for multiple system atrophy? Arch Neurol 1999; **56**: 225–8.

Morrish PK, Sawle GV, Brooks DJ. Clinical and ^{18}F-dopa PET findings in early Parkinson's disease. J Neurol Neurosurg Psychiatry 1995; **59**: 597–600.

Morrish PK, Rakshi JS, Bailey DL, Sawle GV, Brooks DJ. Measuring the rate of progression and estimating the preclinical period of Parkinson's disease with ^{18}F-dopa PET. J Neurol Neurosurg Psychiatry 1998; **64**: 314–9.

Morrish PK, Sawle GV, Brooks DJ. An ^{18}F-dopa PET and clinical study of the rate of progression in Parkinson's disease. Brain 1996; **119**: 585–91.

National Collaborating Centre for Chronic Conditions. Diagnosing Parkinson's disease. In: Parkinson's disease – National clinical guideline for diagnosis and management in primary and secondary care. London: Royal College of Physicians, 2006; 29–48.

Pramstaller PP, Wenning GK, Smith SJM, Beck RO, Quinn NP, Fowler CJ. Nerve conduction studies, skeletal muscle EMG, and sphincter EMG in multiple system atrophy. J Neurol Neurosurg Psychiatry 1995; **58**: 618–21.

Schrag A, Kingsley D, Phatouros C et al. Clinical usefulness of magnetic resonance imaging in multiple system atrophy. J Neurol Neurosurg Psychiatry 1998; **65**: 65–71.

Schulz JB, Skalej M, Wedekind D et al. Magnetic resonance imaging-based volumetry differentiates idiopathic Parkinson's disease from multiple system atrophy and progressive supranuclear palsy. Ann Neurol 1999; **45**: 65–74.

Stocchi F, Carbone A, Inghilleri M et al. Urodynamic and neurophysiological evaluation in Parkinson's disease and multiple system atrophy. J Neurol Neurosurg Psychiatry 1997; **62**: 507–11.

Thomaides TN, Chaudhuri KR, Maule S, Watson L, Marsden CD, Mathias CJ. Growth hormone response to clonidine in central and peripheral primary autonomic failure. Lancet 1992; **340**: 263–6.

Tranchant C, Guiraud-Chaumeil C, Warter JM. Stimulation of growth hormone release with clonidine is not a good test to distinguish Parkinson's disease from multiple system atrophy. Mov Disord 1998; **13 (Suppl 2)**: 197.

Valldeoriola F, Valls-Sole J, Tolosa ES, Marti MJ. Striated anal sphincter denervation in patients with progressive supranuclear palsy. Mov Disord 1995; **10**: 550–5.

6 Medical management – neuroprotection

Neuroprotection trial methodology
Potential neuroprotective agents

Parkinson's disease (PD) is a steadily progressive condition. At present, pharmacotherapy can only provide symptomatic benefit to patients. What is required is an agent that can slow the progression of the disease, so-called neuroprotective therapy, or something that can permanently prevent the death of sick nigrostriatal dopaminergic neurones, so-called neurorescue therapy (Fig. 6.1). By slowing or halting the disease, many of the later motor and non-motor complications of PD will never develop, so patient's quality of life will be much improved and the healthcare costs of the condition will be reduced.

Neurorestoration is an increase in the dopaminergic innervation of the striatum which is achieved by either transplantation of new dopaminergic cells or stimulation of existing cells with a growth factor. Such issues will be considered in the chapter on surgery for PD.

> No agent has been proven to slow disease progression in Parkinson's disease

Finding some form of neuroprotective therapy for PD is what patients often refer to as finding a 'cure' for their condition. Understandably, this is a priority for patients in terms of the research agenda. However, the few trials that have been done in this area have produced no clear evidence that any substance is neuroprotective in PD. Furthermore, these trials have raised serious questions about how trials should be conducted in the future, in particular, which outcome measures should be used.

Neuroprotection trial methodology

Since it is impossible to measure the number of remaining dopaminergic neurones in life, neuroprotection trials in PD must use other

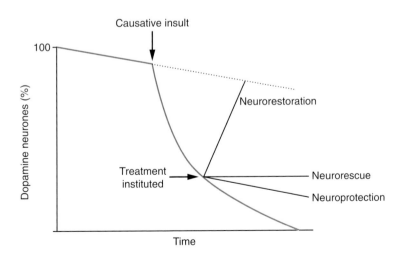

Figure 6.1
Schematic representation of neuroprotection, neurorescue, and neurorestoration in Parkinson's disease therapy.

outcome measures which parallel the number of surviving neurones. A 'surrogate' outcome measure is a physical sign, laboratory measure or investigation which faithfully mirrors clinically meaningful outcomes. We do not know that slowing the loss of dopaminergic neurones in PD is sufficient to be clinically meaningful, so 'surrogate' is not appropriate and the term 'biomarker' is preferred.

> Considerable doubt surrounds the design of neuroprotection trials in Parkinson's disease

Since most of the difficulties with neuroprotection trials in PD have centred on the problems with the existing biomarkers that have been used, it is necessary to discuss these in some detail (Table 6.1), alongside the overall design of neuroprotection trials.

Clinical rating scales

Parallel design trials

The most commonly used clinical rating scale in PD trials over the last 10 years has been the UPDRS (see Table 4.5). Although the total of each part of the UPDRS scale is often used, since patients in the early stages of PD only score on the ADL and motor parts of the scale, the total score is very similar to the sum of the ADL and motor parts of the scale.

In neuroprotection trials, the UPDRS is compared in a group allocated to the active medication with a group given placebo. Provided that the active compound does not have a symptomatic effect in treating the motor features of PD, any difference in UPDRS between placebo and the active preparation should be due to a neuroprotective effect. An example of this type of design is the trial of three different doses of co-enzyme Q_{10} versus placebo (Fig. 6.2). There was a trend to co-enzyme Q_{10} being more effective than placebo which reached statistical significance ($P < 0.05$) for the 1200 mg/day dose.

Parallel design trial with final withdrawal (washout)

The problem with parallel design trials is that it is impossible safely to assume that any

Table 6.1
Relative merits and drawbacks of outcome measures for neuroprotection trials

Outcome measures	Benefits	Problems
Clinical rating scales	Standard method used for many years	Open to symptomatic effects of therapy unless evaluated after drug withdrawal or in delayed start design
Time to end-point	Has direct relevance to people with PD	More likely to be a pharmacokinetic or dynamic effect than neuroprotection
SPECT and PET imaging	Intuitively a good biomarker for the disease May improve diagnostic accuracy at start of trials May be more sensitive than clinical outcomes	People who have PD clinically but have normal baseline scan People with PD with abnormal baseline radionuclide studies may have PSP/MSA Lack of clinical correlation of neuroprotection in imaging studies to date Poor sensitivity to change and reproducibility of radionuclide studies Differential regulation of ligand pharmacokinetics by medication
Mortality	Has direct relevance to people with PD	Open to symptomatic effects of therapy Studies need to be large or long-term to have adequate power
Quality of life	Patient-rated so more meaningful to them	Open to symptomatic effects of therapy Likely to have low sensitivity unless agent has large treatment effect

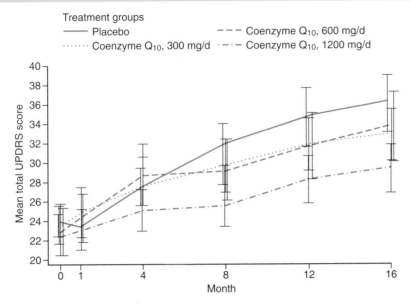

Figure 6.2
Neuroprotection trial comparing three different doses of co-enzyme Q$_{10}$ with placebo in early Parkinson's disease.
Reproduced with permission from: Shultz CW, Oakes D, Kieburtz K *et al*. Effects of coenzyme Q$_{10}$ in early Parkinson disease. *Arch Neurol* 2002; **59**: 1541–50.

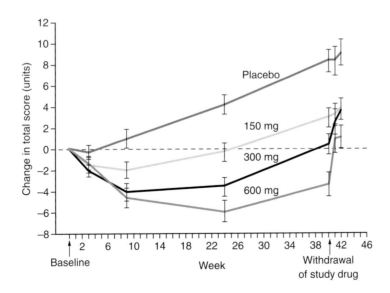

Figure 6.3
Neuroprotection trial comparing three different doses of levodopa (and carbidopa) with placebo in early Parkinson's disease.
Reproduced with permission from: Fahn S, Oakes D, Shoulson I *et al*. and the Parkinson Study Group. Levodopa and the progression of
Parkinson's disease. *N Engl J Med* 2004; **351**: 2498–508.

compound is completely free from any symptomatic effect on PD. To overcome this drawback, a similar parallel design is used, but patients are withdrawn or washed out from all medication at the end of the trial. If the agent under investigation has a symptomatic effect, the UPDRS in the active treatment arm will return to the placebo level. If the agent has had a neuroprotective effect, then the UPDRS will not return to the placebo level. An example of this design is the ELLDOPA trial of three different doses of levodopa versus placebo (Fig. 6.3). The UPDRS declined rapidly when levodopa was withdrawn at the end of the study, but in none of the groups did this reach the placebo level. The problem with this type of design is that PD patients can rarely tolerate withdrawal of symptomatically active medication for very long. So, in the ELLDOPA trial, the 2-week wash-out period was insufficient and with longer, the UPDRS may have reached the placebo level.

Parallel design futility trials

The parallel design neuroprotection trials described above need to be large to find small but significant effects, so they are long and costly. One way to screen compounds for neuroprotective effects more quickly is to perform smaller trials looking for large effects. A systematic programme of trials (Net-PD) has been developed in the US to examine the effects of 12 existing agents which may be neuroprotective. This is funded by the National Institute for Neurologic Diseases and Stroke (NINDS). Agents are being screened in small 'futility studies' looking for a 30% reduction in total UPDRS decline compared with historical control data. If this threshold is not met, agents are likely to be 'futile' as neuroprotectants, so they are not studied further. Successful compounds will go through to larger definitive studies. The first futility study showed that both minocycline and GPI-1485 significantly delay decline in total UPDRS by more than 30%. However, a small placebo comparator group also showed a similar effect, raising doubts about the use of historical controls.

Delayed start design trials

Traditional parallel design trials involve large numbers of patients, with many taking placebo for long periods. The more recent delayed start design trials have the advantage of more patients receiving the potentially neuroprotective agent. They also deal with the problem of additional symptomatic effects of neuroprotective compounds.

The delayed start design is exemplified by the TEMPO trial comparing rasagiline with placebo (Fig. 6.4). In two arms of the trial, patients were commenced on rasagiline, either 1 mg/day or 2 mg/day, at the outset. The UPDRS showed an initial improvement in both groups because of the symptomatic effect of the drug. There was then a steady decline in UPDRS over the following 12 months. The third group of patients were given, in a double-blind fashion, placebo for 6 months followed by rasagiline 2 mg/day. This group showed a small initial improvement, due to a placebo effect. They then deteriorated until rasagiline was commenced at 6 months which led to an improvement before they began to steadily deteriorate again. At the end of the trial, the two groups on 2 mg/day of rasagiline had received symptomatically active drug for 6 months, so one would expect them to have similar UPDRS scores if rasagiline only had a symptomatic effect. However, the UPDRS score was better in the group who had had rasagiline for longer, implying that it had had a neuroprotective effect.

The delayed start design trial is proving very popular at present. However, it still has problems. Sufficiently large numbers of patients are required to ensure differences at the end of the trial are statistically significant; the results in the rasagiline trial (TEMPO) were only just significant at the $P < 0.05$ level, so another larger trial is on-going. Whilst delayed start trials in PD begin with patients who do not need symptomatic therapy, many will develop a need for active treatment over the 12–24 months of the trial. If the trial drug does not have a symptomatic effect, then additional

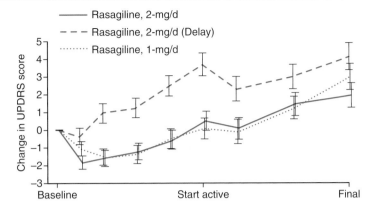

Figure 6.4
Delayed start neuroprotection trial comparing two doses of rasagiline commenced immediately or delayed for 6 months.
Reproduced with permission from: Parkinson Study Group. A controlled, randomized, delayed-start study of rasagiline in early Parkinson disease. *Arch Neurol* 2004; **61**: 561–9.

active medication must be added. There is the potential for bias entering the study if more patients in the delayed start group receive symptomatic therapy than those who have had it all along.

Time to clinical end-point

In this type of neuroprotection trial, the difference in the time to the development of a clinical endpoint is examined. So in the DATATOP trial, the time to the need for symptomatic therapy with levodopa was used as the primary outcome measure; the group randomised to selegiline reached this outcome in smaller numbers than those randomised to placebo (hazard ratio 0.43; 95% CI 0.33, 0.55). However, this trial was confounded by the symptomatic effect of selegiline, so it could not be claimed that the delay in the need for levodopa was due to any neuroprotective effect of selegiline.

It should be noted that delaying the time to onset of any motor complications cannot be attributed to a neuroprotective effect, as this may be due to the levodopa sparing effects of agents, such as dopamine agonists.

Neuroimaging

SPECT and PET scanning can be used to monitor the decline in the dopamine transporter as PD

progresses clinically. Intuitively, this should be an excellent biomarker to use in neuroprotection trials.

Two such studies have been performed. In a 46 months' trial of pramipexole versus levodopa in early PD, the decline in ^{123}I-β-CIT SPECT was less in the patients given pramipexole than those given levodopa (16.0% versus 25.5%; $P = 0.01$). Similarly, in a 2-year trial of ropinirole versus levodopa in early PD, the decline in ^{18}F-fluorodopa PET was less in the patients given ropinirole than those given levodopa (13% versus 20%; $P = 0.022$). The methodology of both of these trials has been heavily criticised (Table 6.1), so the results require confirmation with other trial designs before we can accept that these dopamine agonists are neuroprotective. One of the major concerns was the likelihood that drugs would have a differential effect on dopamine transporter kinetics.

Mortality

Using mortality rate as the primary outcome measure in neuroprotection trials has the advantage of being clinically relevant for patients, but the drawback of requiring large, long-term studies.

The only agent that has undergone wide-spread study using mortality as an outcome is selegiline. Most trials showed no difference in mortality between those given selegiline and those taking placebo. Then the UK Parkinson's Disease Research Group (PDRG) trial found a significant increase in mortality in those given selegiline. This work has recently undergone systematic review (Fig. 6.5), but no significant increase in mortality was found with selegiline (odds ratio 1.13; 95% CI 0.94, 1.34; P = 0.2).

Quality of life

All of the neuroprotection trial outcome measures detailed above, apart from mortality, have the disadvantage that they do not have direct meaning for patients with PD. In theory, using disease-specific, quality-of-life scales (*e.g.* PDQ 39) rated by patients themselves would be more meaningful. However, such trials will need to be very large and long-term and,

to date, such outcomes have not been used as the primary measure.

Potential neuroprotective agents

Discussion of the mechanisms of action of compounds which may be neuroprotective is beyond the scope of this book, but the processes they are likely to interfere with are outlined in Table 6.2.

Table 6.2
Potential sites of action of neuroprotective agents in Parkinson's disease

---

- Mitochondrial complex-1 deficiency
- Free radical damage and oxidative stress
- Proteasomal dysfunction
- Apoptosis
- Inflammation (microglial activation)

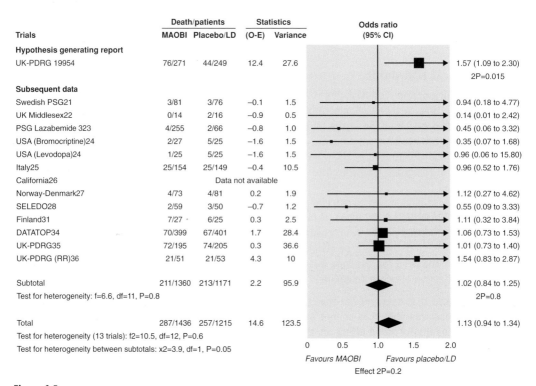

Trials	Death/patients		Statistics		Odds ratio (95% CI)	
	MAOBI	Placebo/LD	(O-E)	Variance		
Hypothesis generating report						
UK-PDRG 19954	76/271	44/249	12.4	27.6		1.57 (1.09 to 2.30)
						2P=0.015
Subsequent data						
Swedish PSG21	3/81	3/76	−0.1	1.5		0.94 (0.18 to 4.77)
UK Middlesex22	0/14	2/16	−0.9	0.5		0.14 (0.01 to 2.42)
PSG Lazabemide 323	4/255	2/66	−0.8	1.0		0.45 (0.06 to 3.32)
USA (Bromocriptine)24	2/27	5/25	−1.6	1.5		0.35 (0.07 to 1.68)
USA (Levodopa)24	1/25	5/25	−1.6	1.5		0.96 (0.06 to 15.80)
Italy25	25/154	25/149	−0.4	10.5		0.96 (0.52 to 1.76)
California26		Data not available				
Norway-Denmark27	4/73	4/81	0.2	1.9		1.12 (0.27 to 4.62)
SELEDO28	2/59	3/50	−0.7	1.2		0.55 (0.09 to 3.33)
Finland31	7/27	6/25	0.3	2.5		1.11 (0.32 to 3.84)
DATATOP34	70/399	67/401	1.7	28.4		1.06 (0.73 to 1.53)
UK-PDRG35	72/195	74/205	0.3	36.6		1.01 (0.73 to 1.40)
UK-PDRG (RR)36	21/51	21/53	4.3	10		1.54 (0.83 to 2.87)
Subtotal	211/1360	213/1171	2.2	95.9		1.02 (0.84 to 1.25)
Test for heterogeneity: f=6.6, df=11, P=0.8						2P=0.8
Total	287/1436	257/1215	14.6	123.5		1.13 (0.94 to 1.34)
Test for heterogeneity (13 trials): f2=10.5, df=12, P=0.6						
Test for heterogeneity between subtotals: x2=3.9, df=1, P=0.05						

0   0.5   1.0   1.5   2.0

Favours MAOBI   *Favours placebo/LD*

Effect 2P=0.2

Figure 6.5
Meta-analysis of trials which examined the mortality rate in Parkinson's disease patients treated with selegiline compared with placebo.
Reproduced with permission from: Ives NJ, Stowe RL, Marro J *et al. BMJ* 2004; **329**: 593–9.

A systematic review of preclinical and clinical neuroprotection trials found a list of 12 compounds that require further clinical neuroprotection trials (Table 6.3). The protective effects of caffeine and nicotine are discussed in Chapter 2 and the early futility studies with minocycline and GPI-1485 earlier in this chapter. The on-going trial with co-enzyme Q_{10} has also been mentioned above. Interest in the neuroprotective properties of monoamine oxidase type B inhibitors is now centred on another delayed start design trial with rasagiline, and further neuroprotection trials are underway with non-ergot dopamine agonists.

Table 6.3
Potential neuroprotective agents in Parkinson's disease

- Caffeine
- Co-enzyme Q_{10}
- Creatine
- GM-1 ganglioside
- GPI-1485
- Minocycline
- Nicotine
- Oestrogen
- Monoamine oxidase inhibitors (rasagiline and selegiline)
- Dopamine agonists (ropinirole and pramipexole)

From Ravina BM, Fagan SC, Hart RG et al. Neuroprotective agents for clinical trials in Parkinson's disease. *Neurology* 2003; **60**: 1234–40.

The pharmaceutical industry is generating many more potential neuroprotectants for neurodegenerative conditions using high throughput models. It is hoped that one or more of these new compounds or older agents will be shown to conclusively slow the progression of PD.

Further reading

Clarke CE, Guttman M. Dopamine agonist monotherapy in Parkinson's disease. *Lancet* 2002; **360**: 1767–9.

Clarke CE. A 'cure' for Parkinson's disease: can neuroprotection be proven with current trial designs? *Mov Disord* 2004; **19**: 491–9.

Clarke CE. Neuroprotection and pharmacotherapy for motor symptoms in Parkinson's disease. *Lancet Neurol* 2004; **3**: 466–75.

Ives N, Stowe R, Marro J et al. Monoamine oxidase B inhibitor therapy in early Parkinson's disease: a systematic review of randomised controlled trials. *BMJ* 2004; **329**: 593–9.

Lees AJ, Parkinson's Disease Research Group of the United Kingdom. Comparison of the therapeutic effects and mortality data of levodopa and levodopa combined with selegiline in patients with early, mild Parkinson's disease. *BMJ* 1995; **311**: 1602–7.

NINDS NET-PD Investigators. A randomized, double-blind, futility clinical trial of creatine and minocycline in early Parkinson disease. *Neurology* 2006; **66**: 664–71.

Parkinson Study Group. A controlled, randomised, delayed-start study of rasagiline in early Parkinson's disease. *Arch Neurol* 2004; **61**: 561–6.

Parkinson Study Group. Effect of deprenyl on the progression of disability in early Parkinson's disease. *N Engl J Med* 1989; **321**: 1364–71.

Parkinson Study Group. Effects of tocopherol and deprenyl on the progression of disability in early Parkinson's disease. *N Engl J Med* 1993; **328**: 176–83.

Parkinson Study Group. Impact of deprenyl and tocopherol treatment on Parkinson's disease in DATATOP patients receiving levodopa. *Ann Neurol* 1996; **39**: 37–45.

Parkinson Study Group. Impact of deprenyl and tocopherol treatment on Parkinson's disease in DATATOP subjects not receiving levodopa. *Ann Neurol* 1996; **39**: 29–36.

Parkinson Study Group. Levodopa and the progression of Parkinson's disease. *N Engl J Med* 2004; **351**: 2498–508.

Parkinson Study Group. Mortality in DATATOP: a multicentre trial in early Parkinson's disease. *Ann Neurol* 1998; **43**: 318–25.

Parkinson Study Group. Pramipexole versus levodopa as initial treatment for Parkinson's disease. *JAMA* 2000; **284**: 1931–8.

Parkinson's Disease Research Group. Comparisons of therapeutic effects of levodopa, levodopa and selegiline, and bromocriptine in patients with early, mild Parkinson's disease: three year interim report. *BMJ* 1993; **307**: 469–72.

Ravina BM, Fagan SC, Hart RG et al. Neuroprotective agents for clinical trials in Parkinson's disease. *Neurology* 2003; **60**: 1234–40.

Shults C, Oakes D, Kieburtz K et al. Effects of coenzyme Q_{10} in early Parkinson disease: evidence of slowing of the functional decline. *Arch Neurol* 2002; **59**: 1541–50.

Whone A, Watts R, Stoessl A et al. Slower progression of Parkinson's disease with ropinirole versus levodopa: the REAL-PET study. *Ann Neurol* 2003; **54**: 93–101.

7 Medical management – symptomatic therapy I: levodopa

Brief history
Pharmacology
Clinical trials
Side-effects
Is levodopa toxic?
Immediate-release levodopa in clinical practice
Modified-release levodopa
Duodenal infusion of levodopa

Brief history

The levodopa story began in 1957 when Carlsson and colleagues demonstrated reversal of akinesia in reserpinised animals following administration of D,L-dopa suggesting a role for dopamine deficiency in Parkinson's disease (PD). Three years later, Ehringer and Hornykiewicz then reported dopamine deficiency in the striatum in PD. In 1961, they found, along with Barbeau, that levodopa treatment had a beneficial effect on motor function in PD in small studies. Dopamine itself does not cross the blood–brain barrier. However, these studies used relatively small doses of levodopa which produced such little benefit that its therapeutic potential was nearly missed. Too much levodopa was being metabolised in the periphery and so the amount delivered to the brain was small. It took until 1967 for Cotzias and colleagues to demonstrate dramatic improvement in motor impairments in PD using larger doses of D,L-dopa in just 17 patients.

The therapeutic potential of levodopa was restricted in these early days by the marked nausea and vomiting it produced. The development of two peripheral dopa decarboxylase inhibitors – carbidopa and benserazide – in the mid-1970s allowed a reduction in the dose of levodopa whilst still allowing large amounts to cross the blood–brain barrier. The development of these dopa decarboxylase inhibitors greatly increased the acceptance of levodopa therapy and reduced the cost. However, prescription rates were slow to increase and it took until the late 1980s for these to plateau in the UK, suggesting that all suitable patients were by then receiving levodopa treatment.

Pharmacology

Levodopa (Fig. 7.1) is absorbed from the small bowel using the large amino acid transport system and is then rapidly distributed with a plasma half life of 60 minutes. It uses the same active transport mechanism to cross the blood–brain barrier. Consequently, gastric emptying and competition from protein in the diet can interfere with absorption and transfer into the brain. Levodopa is metabolised peripherally and centrally by dopa decarboxylase and catechol-O-methyl transferase (COMT) to dopamine and 3-0-methyldopa, respectively (Fig. 7.2).

To reduce the peripheral metabolism of levodopa, it is usually administered with a dopa decarboxylase inhibitor such as carbidopa (Sinemet® or co-careldopa) or benserazide (Madopar® or co-beneldopa). Further peripheral metabolism can be reduced by COMT inhibitors, such as entacapone and tolcapone (chapter 9),

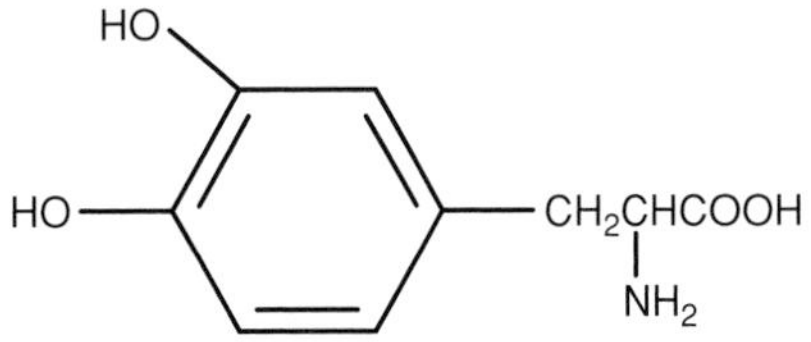

Figure 7.1
Chemical structure of levodopa.

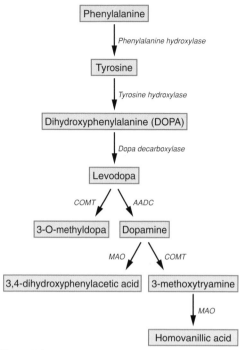

Figure 7.2
Catecholamine biosynthesis and metabolism.

and monoamine oxidase type B (MAOB) inhibitors (chapters 6 and 9). The pharmacokinetic characteristics of the two available modified-release levodopa

preparations and intraduodenal infusion of levodopa are discussed later in this chapter.

As a result of the various combinations of agents and their different doses, a wide range of levodopa preparations are available (Table 7.1). This is confused further by the varied nomenclature used in different countries.

Clinical trials

Levodopa was developed before the age of randomised controlled trials. It can also be argued that, with such a striking clinical effect, few trials would be required. However, some preclinical studies have suggested that levodopa may be toxic, so a recent large randomised controlled trial (ELLDOPA) has finally compared levodopa with placebo. A total of 361 patients were randomised to placebo or three different doses of co-careldopa (Sinemet® 150, 300 and 600 mg/day) for 40 weeks after which the medication was withdrawn for 2 weeks. The total UPDRS score improved with levodopa in a dose-dependent manner (Fig. 7.3) which was significantly better than placebo.

> Levodopa remains the 'gold standard' treatment for Parkinson's disease despite the occurrence of motor complications

Table 7.1
Levodopa preparations available in the UK

Brand name	Generic name	Release mechanism	Levodopa dose (mg)	Decarboxylase dose (mg)
Sinemet® LS (Low Strength)/ Sinemet® 62.5	Co-careldopa	Immediate	50	12.5
Sinemet® 110	Co-careldopa	Immediate	100	10
Sinemet® Plus/Sinemet® 125	Co-careldopa	Immediate	100	25
Sinemet® 275	Co-careldopa	Immediate	250	25
Half Sinemet® CR	Co-careldopa	Modified-release	100	25
Sinemet® CR	Co-careldopa	Modified-release	200	50
Madopar® Dispersible 62.5	Co-beneldopa	Rapid-release	50	12.5
Madopar® Dispersible 125	Co-beneldopa	Rapid-release	100	25
Madopar® 62.5	Co-beneldopa	Immediate	50	12.5
Madopar® 125	Co-beneldopa	Immediate	100	25
Madopar® 250	Co-beneldopa	Immediate	200	50
Madopar® CR	Co-beneldopa	Modified-release	100	25

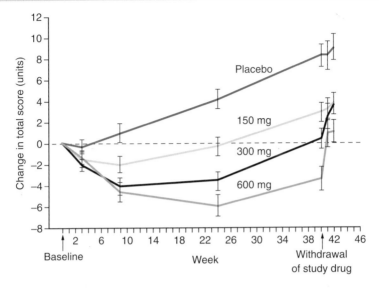

Figure 7.3
ELLDOPA trial comparing three different doses of levodopa (and carbidopa) with placebo in early Parkinson's disease.
Reproduced with permission from: Parkinson Study Group. Levodopa and the progression of Parkinson's disease. *N Engl J Med* 2004; **351:** 2498–508.

A number of studies in the late 1970s compared the two immediate-release levodopa preparations available. Although these trials were small and only medium term (3–6 months), no significant differences in efficacy or adverse events were found between co-careldopa or co-beneldopa.

Side-effects

Short-term side-effects

Many patients suffer initial side-effects when starting levodopa therapy (Table 7.2). The most common are nausea, loss of appetite, and vomiting. Tolerance often develops after several weeks of treatment with complete resolution of symptoms. However, some will require treatment with the only available anti-emetic which does not cross the blood–brain barrier, domperidone (Motilium®; 10–30 mg tid). Postural hypotension can also occur, but this usually settles without the need for treatment. If it does not, then an alternative diagnosis should be considered, commonly multiple system atrophy (MSA; chapter 4).

Sleep disorders triggered by dopaminergic therapy have received little attention in the past, but this has changed after recent concerns about the sudden onset of sleep with

Table 7.2
Short-term side-effects of levodopa

Gastrointestinal
● Nausea
● Vomiting
● Loss of appetite

Cardiovascular
● Postural hypotension

Sleep disorders
● Somnolence
● Insomnia
● Vivid dreams
● Nightmares
● Inversion of sleep–wake cycle

Psychiatric
● Confusion
● Visual hallucinations
● Delusions
● Illusions

dopamine agonists. Levodopa can cause insomnia, vivid dreams, nightmares, somnolence, and an inversion of the sleep–wake cycle. Most of these will resolve with good sleep hygiene and by ensuring that the last dose of levodopa is taken early enough in the evening. Although psychotic adverse events are more commonly seen in later PD, infrequently illusions, visual hallucinations, confusion, and delusions occur with early levodopa treatment. This is more likely if the patient is dementing or with combinations of antiparkinsonian drugs.

Long-term side-effects

As PD progresses, increases in medication are necessary to maintain motor function. Modern practice is to use adjuvant therapies to reduce the dependency on levodopa, otherwise the long-term complications of levodopa can develop sooner than necessary. These complications are comprised of motor and psychiatric side-effects (Table 7.3). The long-term psychiatric side-effects of levodopa, including illusions, visual hallucinations, confusion, and delusions, are considered with the non-motor complications of PD in chapter 10. Motor complications are comprised of abnormal involuntary movements (AIMs) or dyskinesias and response fluctuations.

Table 7.3
Long-term side-effects of levodopa

Involuntary movements
- Peak-dose athetoid dyskinesia
- Diphasic dyskinesia (at start and end of dose)
- Dystonia (painful cramp in foot)

Response fluctuations
- End-of-dose deterioration (wearing off)
- Unpredictable 'on'/'off' switching

Psychiatric
- Confusion
- Visual hallucinations
- Delusions
- Illusions

Abnormal involuntary movements

Abnormal involuntary movements are athetoid or fluid twisting movements of the limbs, trunk, or face. These are usually a peak-dose phenomenon; rarely, they can recur just as the effect of an individual dose wanes, giving rise to diphasic dyskinesia.

The other common AIM is dystonia, in which painful muscle contractions cause unusual postures. This can affect the leg, leading to painful plantar flexion and inversion at the ankle and extension of the great toe (so-called 'striatal toe'). Rarely, it can cause flexion of the fingers into the palm of the hand. These phenomena frequently occur in the early morning. Dystonia occurred in the days prior to levodopa therapy and, thus, can be part of the underlying disease process. The increase in dystonia with levodopa therapy clearly links the two but, paradoxically, dystonia often responds to taking a dose of levodopa for reasons which are not understood.

Response fluctuations

These include a shortening of the response to each dose of levodopa (end-of-dose deterioration or the wearing-off effect) and unpredictable switching between the mobile 'on' phase and the relatively immobile 'off' phase. The latter can occur so rapidly that it resembles the switching on and off of a light switch, a point not often understood by carers and staff.

Prevalence and aetiology of motor complications

Motor complications (Table 7.4) have been shown to occur in 50% of PD patients after 6 years of levodopa therapy and in 100% of young-onset patients (onset < 40 years) after 6 years of treatment. So, motor complications are related to the duration of levodopa therapy and younger patients are more susceptible to them.

In the ELLDOPA trial, dyskinesia developed in 17% of patients on 600 mg/day of levodopa after 40 weeks of treatment, compared with 2% on 300 mg/day, 3% on 150 mg/day and 3% on

Table 7.4
Factors associated with the development of motor complications on levodopa

- Duration of therapy
- Dose
- Severity of disease
- Pulsatile stimulation with immediate-release preparations

Whether patients with early Parkinson's disease should be initiated on levodopa, a non-ergot dopamine agonist or a MAOB inhibitor is unknown but is the subject of the PD MED trial

---

placebo. So, dyskinesia is related to the dose of levodopa used.

The MPTP-treated primate model of PD has more severe loss of dopaminergic neurones than in early PD. These animals develop dose-dependent motor complications within just days or weeks of first receiving levodopa therapy. This implies that the severity of PD also plays a part in the genesis of motor complications.

In view of its short half-life, immediate-release levodopa provides pulsatile stimulation of dopamine receptors. Taking 3–5 levodopa doses per day produces the equivalent number of peaks and troughs in blood and, thus, brain levels of levodopa. Providing continuous dopaminergic stimulation (CDS) with levodopa, apomorphine or lisuride infusions in patients with later PD produces major improvements in motor complications. In early PD, the longer acting dopamine agonists produce fewer and later motor complications than levodopa monotherapy. A trial in early PD patients (STRIDE) is currently examining whether reducing pulsatile stimulation by adding the COMT inhibitor entacapone to co-careldopa reduces motor complications. So, pulsatile stimulation with immediate-release levodopa preparations is involved in the production of motor complications.

Management of motor complications

The management of motor complications is complex and requires considerable experience. The modern approach is to avoid or delay their onset by using initial monotherapy with an alternative to levodopa, such as a dopamine agonist or MAOB inhibitor, although this remains controversial.

The simplest approach to treating motor complications is to fractionate the dose of levodopa. For example, a patient with complications on Sinemet®, 275 tid, may respond better to Sinemet® Plus (125) taken 5 times daily. This reduces the peak effect of levodopa and thus dyskinesia whilst filling in the gaps between the tid regimen so that end-of-dose deterioration is reduced. However, occasionally, this can lead to a sub-threshold dose of levodopa so that the patient never switches 'on'.

The other approach to treating motor complications is adjuvant therapy with a dopamine agonist, COMT inhibitor or MAOB inhibitor (discussed in chapters 8 and 9). Another approach has been to use modified-release preparations of levodopa which are considered later in this chapter.

Is levodopa toxic?

Tissue culture experiments have shown that dopamine and levodopa are both toxic to dopaminergic cells, but this has yet to be demonstrated *in vivo* and in the presence of glial cells. Small postmortem studies of patients without PD who had mistakenly received levodopa for long periods have shown normal dopaminergic cell counts implying that levodopa had not damaged their normal dopamine neurones.

Whether levodopa is toxic in PD patients has been addressed in the recent ELLDOPA Trial. The design of the study has been outlined above. When levodopa was withdrawn for 2 weeks at the end of 40 weeks' treatment, the total UPDRS scores of all of the patients on levodopa fell towards, but did not reach, the level seen in the placebo group (Fig. 7.3). This might imply that levodopa acted as a neuroprotective agent. However, it could also be interpreted as too short a wash-out period, since levodopa is known to have a long-lasting effect, perhaps due to storage in the remaining dopaminergic neurones. A potential neuroprotective effect for levodopa was also unlikely as SPECT scanning in a sub-set of 116 patients showed a significantly greater decline in dopamine transporter uptake with levodopa than placebo.

So, there is insufficient evidence on which to decide whether levodopa is toxic or neuroprotective in PD.

Immediate-release levodopa in clinical practice

Once the decision to use immediate-release levodopa has been taken, it is customary to commence with the smallest dose of levodopa (with a decarboxylase inhibitor) which will control the patient's symptoms. Many patients can tolerate therapeutic doses immediately, such as co-careldopa or co-beneldopa 125 tid, taken with their main meals to reduce gastrointestinal side-effects. However, older or frail patients are best commenced on lower doses (e.g. co-careldopa or co-beneldopa 62.5 tid) which are titrated up gradually towards a therapeutic dose over several weeks. All patients will need to be reviewed by their specialist or Parkinson's Disease Nurse Specialist after 1–2 months of treatment to assess their response and any side-effects. At this stage, a further increase, or even a decrease, in dose may be necessary, or domperidone 10–20 mg tid may be needed to reduce gastrointestinal side-effects. Once stabilised in this way, patients are likely to be receiving co-careldopa or co-beneldopa 62.5 tds to 125 tid, all doses taken with main meals.

As PD progresses, larger doses of levodopa will become necessary to manage motor disabilities. Some clinicians presage the need to fractionate immediate-release levodopa doses as the disease progresses by titrating up to co-careldopa or co-beneldopa 125 taken 5 times daily (i.e. with three main meals and 'mid-morning coffee' and 'mid-afternoon tea').

> The dose of levodopa should be kept at or below around 600 mg/day to reduce the likelihood of motor complications

The ELLDOPA trial has shown that levodopa doses of 600 mg/day lead to dyskinesias with just 40 weeks of therapy in 17% of PD cases. This tends to confirm the modern strategy to keep the dose of levodopa to a maximum of around 500–600 mg/day by adding adjuvant agents before motor complications have developed. There is no direct trial evidence to support this approach; however, some data may come from the on-going PD MED trial.

Modified-release levodopa

Slow- or modified-release preparations of levodopa were originally developed in an effort to overcome the motor fluctuations seen with long-term therapy in later PD. Madopar® CR has a novel release mechanism in which the gelatine shell of the capsule undergoes dissolution when it meets gastric fluid and a mucous body is formed which floats on the surface of the stomach. It remains in the stomach for prolonged periods of time releasing levodopa and benserazide through a hydrated layer by diffusion. The drawback is that its bioavailability after oral dosing is reduced to 60–70% of that of standard Madopar®, due to incomplete absorption rather than altered disposition.

Sinemet® CR differs from its counterpart in being a slowly eroding, polymer-based matrix containing levodopa and carbidopa. In elderly subjects, the bioavailability of levodopa is also reduced with Sinemet® CR to 70% of that of the standard Sinemet®.

Clinical trials in patients with motor complications showed that both modified-release preparations produced moderate reductions in 'off' time, but a slight increase in dyskinesia. Larger doses (20–60%) of the modified-release preparations were required to achieve this effect because of poor absorption. Whilst in these trials, clinicians and patients preferred the modified-release preparations, in standard clinical practice the unpredictability of the response to modified-release levodopa has led to them largely being abandoned.

Two studies have examined the use of modified-release levodopa in early untreated disease in the hope of preventing long-term motor complications. The first of these was a randomised, double-blind, parallel group multicentre study of 134 Danish-Norwegian patients with untreated *de novo* PD randomised to Madopar® CR or standard Madopar®. After 5 years, there was no difference in the frequency of motor fluctuations (57% Madopar® CR versus 59% standard Madopar®) or dyskinesia (34% Madopar® CR versus 41% standard Madopar®). The analogous trial with Sinemet® CR (CR First Study) was a randomised, triple-blind (*i.e.* statistical analysis was also performed blind), parallel group design in 35 centres world-wide. A total of 618 untreated patients were randomised. After 5 years, there was no difference in motor fluctuations between those receiving standard Sinemet® and those on Sinemet® CR (16% in both groups). The low incidence of fluctuations compared with other studies was due to the strict criteria used to define the presence of fluctuations in this trial.

In conclusion, modified-release levodopa preparations are no better than immediate-release levodopa with regard to the genesis of motor complications, so there is no justification in using these more expensive agents in *de novo* PD.

> Modified-release levodopa preparations are of little value to prevent motor complications in early Parkinson's disease or to treat them once they have developed in later Parkinson's disease. They should be restricted to treating nocturnal hypokinesia

However, one valuable place for modified-release levodopa is in patients with nocturnal hypokinesia. This can produce significant improvement in mobility throughout the night, allowing patients to turn in bed more freely and reach the toilet without the assistance of a carer. There can also be beneficial effects left by the following morning so that the patient has a longer period of sleep benefit. Large doses must be avoided as these can produce nightmares, confusion and/or hallucinations.

Duodenal infusion of levodopa

Once severe motor complications have developed on levodopa and multiple adjuvant therapies in very advanced PD, the limited therapeutic options include replacement of some or all oral therapy with either an apomorphine infusion (chapter 8) or bilateral subthalamic stimulation (chapter 11).

Recently, an alternative has been licensed in which a levodopa gel (Duodopa®) is infused directly into the duodenum to provide CDS (Figs 7.4 and 7.5). Small cross-over trials have shown that intraduodenal levodopa gel infusions can

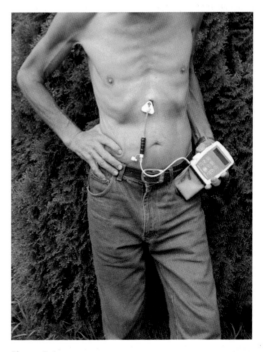

Figure 7.4
Patient undergoing levodopa gel (Duodopa®) infusion.

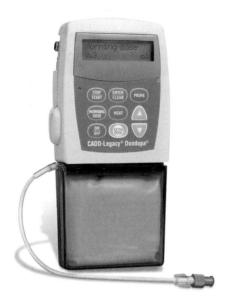

Figure 7.5
Control system for levodopa gel (Duodopa®) infusion.

reduce 'off' periods and improve UPDRS motor and ADL scores, along with quality-of-life ratings.

However, although this technique can be commenced through a nasogastric tube, it eventually requires percutaneous gastrostomy. This can be hazardous in debilitated patients with advanced PD and there can be problems with the tube becoming dislodged and needing to be replaced. It is estimated that the cost of intraduodenal levodopa infusion is around £30,000 per annum per patient which compares with around £10,000 per annum for apomorphine infusion and £6,000 per annum for bilateral subthalamic deep brain

stimulation. It should, therefore, be restricted to PD patients who are not fit for surgery or apomorphine infusion and preferably those who cannot take medication orally because of upper gastrointestinal tract pathology.

Further reading

Block G, Liss C, Reines S, Irr J, Nibbelink D, Group TCFS. Comparison of immediate-release and controlled-release carbidopa/levodopa in Parkinson's disease. *Eur Neurol* 1997; **37**: 23–7.

Clarke CE. Modified-release drugs for Parkinson's disease. *Prescriber* 1997; **8**: 85–90.

Clarke CE. Neuroprotection and pharmacotherapy for motor symptoms in Parkinson's disease. *Lancet Neurol* 2004; **3**: 466–75.

Cotzias GC, Woert MHV, Schiffer LM. Aromatic amino acids and modification of parkinsonism. *N Engl J Med* 1967; **276**: 374–9.

Dupont E, Anderson A, Boas J *et al*. Sustained-release Madopar® HBS compared with standard Madopar® in the long-term treatment of *de novo* parkinsonian patients. *Acta Neurol Scand* 1996; **93**: 14–20.

National Collaborating Centre for Chronic Conditions. Symptomatic pharmacological therapy in Parkinson's disease. In: *Parkinson's disease – National clinical guideline for diagnosis and management in primary and secondary care*. London: Royal College of Physicians, 2006; 59–99.

Nyholm D, Nilsson Remahl AIM, Dizdar N *et al*. Duodenal levodopa infusion monotherapy versus polypharmacy in advanced Parkinson's disease. *Neurology* 2005; **64**: 216–23.

Olanow CW, Obeso JA, Stocchi F. Continuous dopamine-receptor treatment of Parkinson's disease: scientific rationale and clinical implications. *Lancet Neurol* 2006; **5**: 677–87.

Parkinson Study Group. Levodopa and the progression of Parkinson's disease. *N Engl J Med* 2004; **351**: 2498–508.

PD MED website <http://www.pdmed.bham.ac.uk>.

Quinn N, Critchley P, Parkes D, Marsden CD. When should levodopa be started? *Lancet* 1986; **ii**: 985–6.

8 Medical management – symptomatic therapy II: dopamine agonists

Brief history
Pharmacology
Titration and adverse effects
Dopamine agonists in early
    Parkinson's disease
Dopamine agonists in later Parkinson's
    disease

Brief history

The first oral dopamine agonists entered clinical practice in the late 1970s. Dopamine agonists act directly on postsynaptic dopamine receptors in the striatum without the need to be converted into dopamine, as does levodopa (chapter 7). They, therefore, bypass the degenerating nigrostriatal dopaminergic neurones, so it was hoped that they would prove more effective than levodopa in the later stages of Parkinson's disease (PD) and perhaps

be better tolerated. Correspondingly, the initial work with the older agonists, such as bromocriptine, was as adjuvant or add-on therapy in patients with motor complications.

Later studies with the older agonists raised the possibility that dopamine agonist monotherapy in the early stages of the disease produces fewer motor complications than levodopa. This led to large, long-term monotherapy trials with the newer agonists with considerable success in reducing motor complications.

Recent concerns about the long-term side-effects of the older ergot-derived dopamine agonists have caused a dramatic decline in their usage in favour of the non-ergot agonists, so these are the focus of this chapter.

Pharmacology

The basic pharmacology of the dopamine agonists which are licensed in the UK are summarised in Table 8.1. Recently, a non-ergot dopamine agonist, rotigotine, has become available in a transdermal delivery system which provides 24-hour dopaminergic stimulation. This will be considered with the other non-ergot agonists. The parenterally administered dopamine agonist apomorphine will be considered separately in view of its unique characteristics and use in later PD.

There are two groups of dopamine receptor – the D_2 and the D_1 receptor 'families' (Fig. 8.1).

Table 8.1
Basic pharmacology of dopamine agonists

Agonist	D_2 group affinity	D_1 group affinity	Ergot-derived	$t_{1/2}$ (h)	t_{max} (h)	Clearance
Bromocriptine	+++	−	Yes	3–6	1.2	Hepatic metabolism
Cabergoline	+++	0	Yes	65	0.5–4.0	Hepatic metabolism
Lisuride	++	0/−	Yes	2–3	1.0	Hepatic metabolism
Pergolide	+++	+	Yes	15–42	2.0	Renal excretion
Pramipexole	+++	0	No	8–12	1–3	Renal excretion (90%)
Ropinirole	+++	0	No	3–5	1–2	Hepatic metabolism
Rotigotine	+++	++	No	24-h stimulation by patch		Multiple*
Apomorphine	+++	+++	No	0.5	8 min	Hepatic metabolism

+, agonist; −, antagonist; 0/−, partial antagonist; *glucuronidation, sulphation and N-dealkylation.

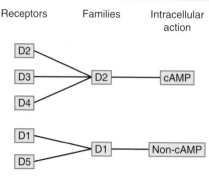

Figure 8.1
Dopamine receptor subtypes. cAMP, cyclic adenosine monophosphate.

Titration and adverse effects

The side-effect profiles of the dopamine agonists are similar to those of levodopa but such problems occur more frequently and/or with greater severity. The most commonly experienced are shown in Table 8.2. Most of these can be avoided by slow titration of the agonist. Tables 8.3–8.5 give details of the titration regimens of the commonly used non-ergot agonists which should be of value in clinical practice.

Gastrointestinal problems and some postural hypotension can be blocked with the peripheral dopamine D_2 receptor antagonist domperidone (10–20 mg tid). Tolerance to these dopaminergic effects usually develops over several weeks of treatment.

> Non-ergot dopamine agonists should now be initiated instead of ergot-derived agonists to avoid serosal reactions and cardiac valvulopathy

Ergot-derived agonists can cause their own specific problems such as ankle oedema, erythromelalgia (*i.e.* florid erythema and swelling of the lower limb), and Raynaud's phenomenon. Rarely, serosal complications such as retroperitoneal, pericardial and pleural effusions and/or fibrosis are seen with dopamine agonists. It is generally thought that these are more common with ergot-derived

Table 8.2
Common side-effects of dopamine agonists

- Nausea, vomiting, loss of appetite
- Postural hypotension
- Confusion, hallucinations
- Somnolence

Table 8.3
Ropinirole titration regimen

Week 1	Starter pack	0.25 mg tid
Week 2	Starter pack	0.5 mg tid
Week 3	Starter pack	0.75 mg tid
Week 4	Starter pack	1 mg tid
Week 5	Follow-on pack	1.5 mg tid
Week 6	Follow-on pack	2 mg tid
Week 7	Follow-on pack	2.5 mg tid
Week 8	Follow-on pack	3 mg tid
Week 9	Standard prescribing	4 mg tid
Week 10	Standard prescribing	5 mg tid
Week 11	Standard prescribing	6 mg tid
Week 12	Standard prescribing	7 mg tid
Week 13	Standard prescribing	8 mg tid

Initial therapeutic range: monotherapy 8–12 mg/day; adjuvant therapy 12–24 mg/day.

Table 8.4
Pramipexole titration regimen (as hydrochloride salt)

Week 1	0.125 mg tid
Week 2	0.25 mg tid
Week 3	0.5 mg tid
Week 4	0.75 mg tid
Week 5	1 mg tid
Week 6	1.25 mg tid
Week 7	1.5 mg tid

Initial therapeutic range: 1.5–3.0 mg/day; adjuvant therapy 3.0–4.5 mg/day.

Table 8.5
Rotigotine patch titration regimen

Week 1	2 mg/24 h
Week 2	4 mg/24 h
Week 3	6 mg/24 h
Week 4	8 mg/24 h

Initial therapeutic range: 6–8 mg/day, early disease licence only.

agonists, but the number of patient years of experience with the non-ergot agonists is insufficient to be sure that these do not cause similar problems. Recently, several case series have described cardiac valvulopathy with the ergot agonist pergolide.

As a result of these findings, in 2005 the UK Medicines and Healthcare Products Regulatory Agency (MHRA) approved a change to the pergolide *Summary of Product Characteristics* (SPC) which stated that: 'Pergolide should be used second-line after a non-ergot dopamine agonist'. This was echoed in the recent UK National Institute for Health and Clinical Excellence (NICE) guidelines for the diagnosis and management of PD which stated in one recommendation: 'If an ergot-derived dopamine agonist is used, the patient should have a minimum of renal function tests, erythrocyte sedimentation rate (ESR) and chest radiograph performed before starting treatment, and annually thereafter... In view of the monitoring required with ergot-derived dopamine agonists, a non-ergot derived agonist should be preferred in most cases.'

Dopamine agonists in early Parkinson's disease

Orally administered dopamine agonists

After the value of dopamine agonists was demonstrated in adjuvant therapy trials, work turned to assessing their ability in early PD to prevent motor complications by acting as: (i) sole therapy without any levodopa (monotherapy); and (ii) levodopa-sparing agents in combination therapy with levodopa.

After several encouraging trials with bromocriptine and one with lisuride, the manufacturers of the latest dopamine agonists set up long-term monotherapy trials comparing dopamine agonists with levodopa in early PD. The results of all of these trials have been summarised in the recent NICE guidelines and a Cochrane systematic review is underway by a group in the University of Birmingham Clinical Trials Unit. The evidence shows that dopamine

agonists compared with levodopa can delay the development of dyskinesia, dystonia and motor fluctuations. However, dopamine agonists are not as effective in treating the motor features of PD. The agonists also cause many dopaminergic adverse events, although low withdrawal rates suggest that these are mild and often settle over time. The final drawback of dopamine agonists is that they are more expensive than levodopa.

> Non-ergot dopamine agonists can be used as initial monotherapy for PD instead of levodopa

The delay in the onset of dyskinesia with dopamine agonists is typified by the ropinirole versus levodopa trial. In this double-blind trial, 268 patients with early PD were randomised to either ropinirole monotherapy to which levodopa could be added later as 'rescue' treatment ($n = 179$) or levodopa alone with potential levodopa rescue ($n = 89$). After 5 years, only 20% of those in the ropinirole arm had dyskinesia compared with 46% in the levodopa arm (hazard ratio 3.8; 95% CI 2.1, 6.9; $P < 0.0001$; Fig. 8.2). However, at the 5-year time point, UPDRS ADL (part II; Fig. 8.3) and motor (part III) scores were worse in those given ropinirole.

> The relative merits of starting PD patients on a dopamine agonist or levodopa require further evaluation in large pragmatic trials

The ability of dopamine agonist monotherapy to delay the onset of motor complications has led to a strategy of initiating agonist therapy rather than levodopa, at least in young patients. However, many questions remain about this policy and a large trial (PD MED) is on-going in the UK with the hope of clarifying the situation. In the early disease randomisation of PD MED, 750–1000 PD patients are being randomised to any levodopa preparation, any dopamine agonist, or any MAOB inhibitor. The primary outcome measures are patient-rated quality of life (PDQ 39 and EuroQol scales) and health

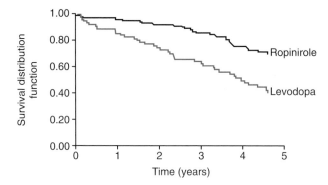

Figure 8.2

Rate of development of dyskinesia in patients with initial ropinirole monotherapy versus levodopa monotherapy.

Reproduced with permission from: Rascol O, Brooks D, Korczyn A, De Deyn P, Clarke C, Lang A. Early treatment with ropinirole reduces the risk of dyskinesia in Parkinson's disease: a 5-year randomised levodopa-controlled study. *N Engl J Med* 2000; **342**: 1484–91.

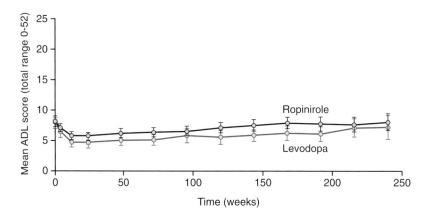

Figure 8.3

UPDRS ADL scores for patients randomised to initial ropinirole monotherapy or levodopa monotherapy (mean and 2SE bars).

Reproduced with permission from: Rascol O, Brooks D, Korczyn A, De Deyn P, Clarke C, Lang A. Early treatment with ropinirole reduces the risk of dyskinesia in Parkinson's disease: a 5-year randomised levodopa-controlled study. *N Engl J Med* 2000; **342**: 1484–91.

economics. This will allow a class effect comparison between agonists and levodopa in terms of quality of life and healthcare costs. As a pragmatic 'real-life' trial, PD MED is randomising older patients than usually enter PD trials, so the results should be more generalisable to everyday practice.

Rotigotine transdermal patch

Recently, a highly lipophilic, non-ergot, dopamine agonist called rotigotine has been formulated into a transdermal patch and licensed for the treatment of early PD. The rotigotine patch produces very stable blood levels over the whole 24-hour period that each patch is used. In theory, such continuous dopaminergic stimulation (CDS) should lead to fewer motor complications than levodopa, but no long-term head-to-head trials have been done against levodopa.

Two placebo-controlled trials have documented the efficacy of rotigotine in improving UPDRS motor and ADL scores in early PD. A further 6-month placebo-controlled trial also had an oral ropinirole comparator arm. Whilst rotigotine was superior to placebo, rotigotine was **not** 'non-inferior' to ropinirole (Fig. 8.4). This occurred because the double-blind titration of ropinirole led to many patients receiving doses of 18–24 mg/day which is much higher than usual for early disease patients. It appears that the current licence maximum 8 mg/day dose of rotigotine is comparable to around 12 mg/day ropinirole. This carries the implication that when patients require titration of medication to doses higher than this, with rotigotine unlicensed levels of 12 to 16 mg/day will be required, compared with ropinirole where 12–24 mg/day doses are available within its current licence.

Choice of dopamine agonist in early Parkinson's disease

The move away from using ergot-derived dopamine agonists, because of concerns about long-term side-effects, has led to increasing use of the non-ergot agonists, pramipexole, ropinirole and, now, rotigotine. Critical appraisal of the literature on the two oral agonists does not provide any evidence-base to prefer one over the other. Oral, once daily, prolonged-release versions of both pramipexole and ropinirole are in development and will compete with the once daily application of the rotigotine patch.

Dopamine agonists in later Parkinson's disease
Orally administered dopamine agonists

The initial trials with oral dopamine agonist therapy were carried out in patients on levodopa who had developed motor complications. The aims of such adjuvant treatment are to:

- reduce the amount of time the patient spends in the relatively immobile 'off' phase

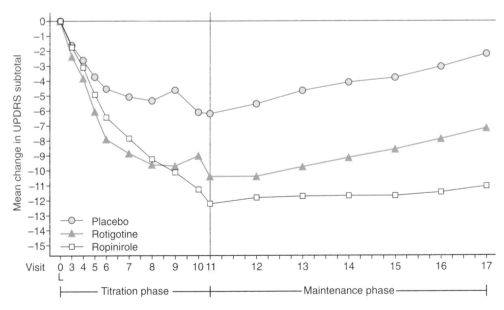

Figure 8.4
Trial of rotigotine patch versus oral ropinirole versus placebo showing beneficial effect of both active drugs compared with placebo but not 'non-inferiority' of rotigotine to ropinirole with the doses used in the study.
Reproduced from rotigotine dossier on EMEA website <http://www.emea.europa.eu>.

- reduce the dose of levodopa in the hope of reducing motor complications in the future and to reduce the side-effects of dopaminergic therapy
- improve motor impairments, disability, and handicap.

These aims should be achieved with an acceptable short-term increase in dyskinesia and other adverse events which can usually be reduced by lowering of the levodopa dose.

> In patients on levodopa who have developed motor complications, adjuvant dopamine agonist therapy can reduce 'off' time, reduce levodopa dose, and reduce motor impairments, but at the expense of increased dyskinesia and other dopaminergic adverse events

The plethora of randomised, controlled trials in this area has undergone systematic review by the Cochrane Movement Disorders Collaborative Review Group. A valuable synthesis of the data on all of the agonists available in the UK is now available electronically on the Cochrane Library. The reviews of placebo-controlled trials show that, in patients already established on levodopa who have developed motor complications, adjuvant dopamine agonist therapy can reduce 'off' time, reduce levodopa dose, and reduce motor impairments, but at the expense of more dyskinesia and other adverse events including nausea, hallucinations, and somnolence. In spite of these side-effects, all-cause withdrawal rates were significantly lower in those given dopamine agonists.

There have also been Cochrane systematic reviews of the adjuvant therapy trials which have compared the more modern agonists with bromocriptine. No clinically worthwhile differences were found.

Choice of dopamine agonist in later Parkinson's disease

There is no evidence to support choosing one dopamine agonist over another in the management of later PD. However, the move towards using non-ergot agonists to avoid long-term side-effects has also occurred in adjuvant therapy. There is no data on which to base a decision between using pramipexole or ropinirole at this stage of the disease.

Apomorphine

Brief history

Apomorphine is an extremely potent D_1 and D_2 dopamine agonist which was used for many years as an emetic. Its bioavailability is poor after oral administration because of extensive first-pass metabolism in the liver. Large doses were used in early studies such that the induced emesis caused pre-renal failure and the cessation of further trials.

Its role as a therapy in PD was developed in London in the late 1980s by Professor Andrew Lees and Dr Gerald Stern. This was facilitated by the availability of the anti-emetic domperidone which, in doses of 10–30 mg tid, can prevent most gastrointestinal problems caused by apomorphine. Subcutaneous bolus doses or continuous infusions of apomorphine were effective in reversing 'off' periods, even in patients with severe fluctuations in response, with a latency of 10–15 minutes. These and most subsequent studies were non-randomised and uncontrolled, but more recent placebo-controlled studies have confirmed the benefits of intermittent apomorphine injections. Continuous infusion of apomorphine costs around £10,000/patient/year, but no health economics' analysis of this costly treatment has been performed. However, the beneficial effects in controlling severe motor fluctuations are such that other costs are likely to be offset, most importantly nursing home placement.

> Intermittent injections of apomorphine can reverse 'off' periods for short periods until oral medication takes effect. For patients with many 'off' periods per day, continuous apomorphine infusion can be a very effective treatment.

Clinical use

Apomorphine therapy is only suitable for use in specialised centres with experience in the technique and usually with a Parkinson's Disease Nurse Specialist (PDNS; chapter 12).

1. The patient is admitted for an acute apomorphine challenge test under domperidone cover, often performed by the nurse.
2. In the 'off' phase, the patient is given an initial dose of around 1 mg apomorphine subcutaneously, escalating at 30-minute intervals through 2, 3, 4, and 6 mg if necessary until a response is seen in motor impairments, which is measured by timed tests of motor function (*e.g.* tapping on two spots 30 cm apart 20 times).
3. Once the threshold dose (usually 2–4 mg) has been established, patients with 5 or 6 'off' periods per day will be given the same number of bolus apomorphine injections just above this dose at the onset of their 'off' periods.
4. If successful in reducing 'off' time, the patient is trained to use a special Penject injection system (Fig. 8.5) which simplifies the process by being pre-filled with apomorphine and having a dial which allows the dose to be easily chosen.

Subcutaneous infusions of apomorphine are used for patients with so many 'off' periods that repeated single dose injections are inappropriate. The drug is drawn up once or twice daily and placed in a portable syringe driver (Fig. 8.5). This is connected to a butterfly cannula which is sited once daily in the abdominal wall or subcutaneous tissue of the thighs. The pump can be programmed to deliver in the range of 50–120 mg of apomorphine over either the waking day or even the whole 24-hour period. The patient's oral medication can then be reduced according to their response. Many are able to withdraw oral agonists and to reduce their levodopa dose substantially. The 'fine tuning' required with this technique is difficult without the benefit of a PDNS who can visit the patient at home. Continuous infusions are not without hazard. The most common is injection site reactions with the oxidised apomorphine irritating the overlying skin causing large bruises and pain (Fig. 8.6). Regular rotation of infusion sites and ultrasonic stimulation can help this problem.

More recently, the intensive use of continuous 'waking day' apomorphine infusions in patients with severe dyskinesia has shown that it can reduce dyskinesia by 65% in severity and 85% in frequency and duration. This suggests that it is an alternative to invasive surgery in such patients.

> A Parkinson's Disease Nurse Specialist is crucial in monitoring apomorphine therapy

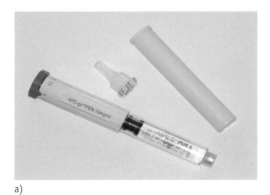

a)

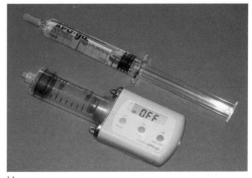

b)

Figure 8.5
(A) Apomorphine Penject injection system; (B) infusion pump with pre-filled syringe.

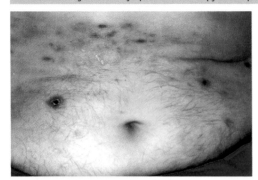

Figure 8.6
Infusion site reaction with apomorphine.

The need for the parenteral administration of apomorphine makes it impractical for many patients. Attempts are underway to create more acceptable delivery methods such as intranasal, sublingual, transdermal, and rectal routes.

Further reading

Clarke CE, Guttman M. Dopamine agonist monotherapy in Parkinson's disease. *Lancet* 2002; **360**: 1767–9.

Clarke CE. Neuroprotection and pharmacotherapy for motor symptoms in Parkinson's disease. *Lancet Neurol* 2004; **3**: 466–75.

Cochrane Library via the Cochrane Collaboration website: <http://www.cochrane.org>.

Colzi A, Turner K, Lees AJ. Continuous subcutaneous waking day apomorphine in the long-term treatment of levodopa-induced interdose dyskinesias in Parkinson's disease. *J Neurol Neurosurg Psychiatry* 1998; **64**: 573–6.

Committee on Safety of Medicines. Fibrotic reactions with pergolideand other ergot-derived dopamine receptor agonists. *Current Problems in Pharmacovigilance* 2002; **28**: 3.

Cotzias G, Papavasiliou P, Tolosa ES *et al*. Treatment of Parkinson's disease with apomorphine: possible role of growth hormone. *N Engl J Med* 1976; **294**: 567–72.

Frankel JP, Lees AJ, Kempster PA, Stern GM. Subcutaneous apomorphine in the treatment of Parkinson's disease. *J Neurol Neurosurg Psychiatry* 1990; **53**: 96–101.

Hutton JT, Dewey RB, LeWitt PA, Factor SA. A randomised double-blind placebo-controlled trial of subcutaneously injected apomorphine for parkinsonian off states. *Mov Disord* 2000; **15 (Suppl 3)**: 130.

National Collaborating Centre for Chronic Conditions. Symptomatic pharmacological therapy in Parkinson's disease. In: *Parkinson's disease – National clinical guideline for diagnosis and management in primary and secondary care*. London: Royal College of Physicians, 2006; 59–99.

Parkinson Study Group. A controlled trial of rotigotine monotherapy in early Parkinson's disease. *Arch Neurol* 2003; **60**: 1721–8.

Parkinson Study Group. Pramipexole versus levodopa as initial treatment for Parkinson's disease: a 4-year randomised controlled trial. *Arch Neurol* 2004; **61**: 1044–53.

PD MED website: <http://www.pdmed.bham.ac.uk>.

Rascol O, Brooks D, Korczyn A, De Deyn P, Clarke C, Lang A. Early treatment with ropinirole reduces the risk of dyskinesia in Parkinson's disease: a 5-year randomised levodopa-controlled study. *N Engl J Med* 2000; **342**: 1484–91.

Shoulson I. Pramipexole versus levodopa in early Parkinson's disease: the randomised controlled CALM-PD trial. *Mov Disord* 2000; **15 (Suppl 3)**: 4.

Van Camp G, Flamez A, Cosyns B *et al*. Treatment of Parkinson's disease with pergolide and relation to restrictive valvular heart disease. *Lancet* 2004; **363**: 1179–83.

9 Medical management – symptomatic therapy III: other therapies

COMT inhibitors
MAOB inhibitors
Amantadine
β-Adrenergic antagonists
Anticholinergics

Catechol-O-methyl transferase (COMT) inhibitors

Pharmacology

By blocking the metabolism of levodopa by the enzyme aromatic amino acid decarboxylase (AADC), predominantly in the gut wall,

benserazide and carbidopa increase the bioavailability of levodopa 2–3-fold and reduce peripheral side-effects in Parkinson's disease (PD). Despite the co-administration of an AADC inhibitor, only 5–10% of the orally administered levodopa crosses the blood–brain barrier. Much of the rest is metabolised to 3-O-methyldopa by the enzyme catechol-O-methyltransferase (COMT) which was first described in 1958. It was hypothesised that blocking the actions of both COMT and AADC might further increase the bioavailability of levodopa (Fig. 7.3).

The first generation of COMT inhibitors appeared in the 1960s and included pyrogallol, tropolones, and 3,4-dihydroxy-2-methylpropiophenone (U-0521). These compounds suffered from weak or non-selective activity, poor bioavailability, or high toxicity, but some did show promising enhancement of the effects of levodopa in animal models.

In 1989, the structure of the second generation of COMT inhibitors was first published by several groups (Fig. 9.1). These di-substituted nitrocatechols do not act in the gut to increase

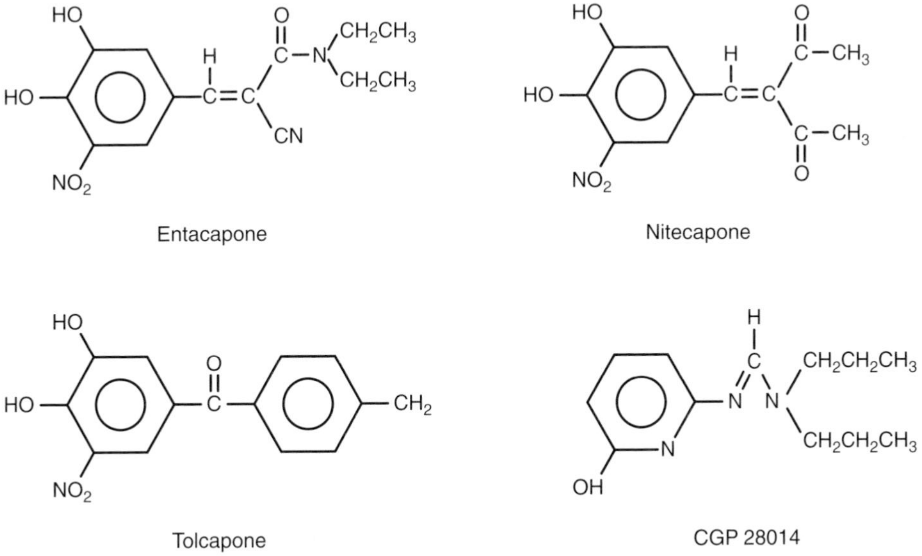

Figure 9.1
Chemical structure of the second generation COMT inhibitors.

levodopa absorption. They seem to have a number of peripheral effects on levodopa metabolism resulting in a 30–50% increase in levodopa half-life and a 25–100% increase in the levodopa concentration versus time curve (area under the curve, AUC), but they do not increase the maximum plasma concentration of levodopa. More levodopa is, therefore, available for longer to cross the blood–brain barrier to produce a more prolonged effect. Tolcapone also has a central effect which may at least in part account for its greater clinical efficacy.

The clinical pharmacology of the second generation COMT inhibitors is summarised in Table 9.1.

Tolcapone

Tolcapone was the first COMT inhibitor to be licensed for use in PD in the UK. Despite promising clinical trial results, tolcapone had to be withdrawn from European Commission countries in November 1998 after the reporting of six cases of hepatitis, three of which were fulminant and ultimately fatal. However, after re-assuring monitoring studies in North America and a switch study suggesting that tolcapone was more effective than entacapone, it was re-introduced to Europe in 2005. The new wording of the tolcapone licence means that it can only be used:

● if entacapone has failed
● at the lower dose of 100 mg tid
● provided appropriate monitoring of liver function is done (2-weekly for 1 year, 4-weekly for next 6 months, 8-weekly

thereafter) with the treatment stopped if enzymes rise 2–3 times above the upper limit of normal.

> Inhibition of COMT with entacapone and tolcapone prolongs the effect of each dose of levodopa thereby reducing 'off' time and allowing a reduction in levodopa dose

Clinical trials

A Cochrane systematic review showed that tolcapone provided a statistically significant reduction in 'off' time in six, randomised, placebo-controlled trials in 1006 patients (100 mg tid dose; weighted means difference on tolcapone minus placebo 1.53 h; 95% CI 0.90, 2.16; $P < 0.00001$). There was a corresponding increase in 'on' time (1.80 h; 95% CI 1.12, 2.48; $P < 0.00001$). A significant reduction in levodopa dose could be achieved with tolcapone (156 mg/day; 95% CI 120, 191; $P < 0.00001$). Few placebo-controlled trials demonstrated benefits in UPDRS ADL or motor scores with tolcapone.

Tolcapone generated typical dopaminergic adverse events, including dyskinesia, nausea and vomiting. Diarrhoea was an unexpected side-effect which necessitated withdrawal in a significant number of patients. The reason for the diarrhoea remains unknown. During clinical trials, an increase in ALT was found in only 1.7% of patients at the 100 mg tid dose. It also caused intensification in the yellow colour of the urine.

Table 9.1
Clinical pharmacology of entacapone and tolcapone

Drug	Structure	Sites of action	t_{max} (h)	$t_{1/2}$ (h)	Dose frequency	Tablet doses (mg)	Clinical dose range (mg/day)
Entacapone	Nitrocatechol	Peripheral	0.4–0.9	0.3–0.4 (α), 1.6–3.4 (β)*	With every levodopa dose tid	200	400–1200
Tolcapone	Nitrocatechol	Peripheral & central	0.9–2.0	2.0–3.0	tid	100	300

*Two-phase model for elimination.

The two trials which compared tolcapone directly with the dopamine agonists bromocriptine and pergolide have been the subject of a Cochrane review, but the trials were insufficiently powered to find differences between the drug classes. Further work is required to compare adjuvant classes to provide guidance on which to choose (*e.g.* PD MED trial).

> COMT inhibitors cause dopaminergic side-effects along with diarrhoea and yellow discolouration of urine

Entacapone

A Cochrane systematic review of eight, randomised, placebo-controlled trials in 1560 patients showed that entacapone leads to statistically significant reduction in 'off' time (weighted means difference on entacapone minus placebo 0.68 h; 95% CI 0.22, 1.13; $P < 0.004$). 'On' time also increased (1.01 h; 95% CI 0.62, 1.39; $P < 0.00001$). Entacapone also led to a significant reduction in levodopa dose (55 mg/day; 95% CI 37, 74; $P < 0.00001$). Some placebo-controlled trials demonstrated small benefits in UPDRS ADL or motor scores with entacapone.

Entacapone produced similar dopaminergic adverse events to tolcapone, including dyskinesia, nausea and vomiting. Diarrhoea was also reported and it caused intensification in the yellow colour of the urine.

> Tolcapone can only be used if entacapone fails, at the dose of 100 mg tid and provided appropriate monitoring of liver function is done (2-weekly for 1 year, 4-weekly for next 6 months, 8-weekly thereafter) with the treatment stopped if enzymes rise 2–3 times above the upper limit of normal

To simplify the use of entacapone with levodopa and carbidopa, a triple combination tablet containing all three drugs is now available (Stalevo®). This has been shown to be popular with patients and may improve compliance which is known to be a problem in PD.

Trials in MPTP-treated marmosets have shown that using entacapone combined with levodopa and carbidopa leads to less dyskinesia than when the same dose of levodopa and carbidopa are used on their own. It is presumed that entacapone increases the trough levels of levodopa and thus provides more continuous dopaminergic stimulation. An analogous clinical trial (STRIDE) is now underway comparing the strategies of initiating therapy with Stalevo® compared with Sinemet®.

Monoamine oxidase type B (MAOB) inhibitors
Selegiline
Pharmacology

Selegiline is a propargylamine which irreversibly inhibits monoamine oxidase type B (MAOB), so it does not cause a tyramine or 'cheese' reaction like the non-selective inhibitors used to treat bipolar depressive disorder. By this inhibition, it reduces the breakdown of dopamine (Fig. 7.3), so more is left in the synaptic cleft. It is metabolised to amphetamine derivatives, so it can have an alerting effect, especially at night, and can have a positive effect in depression. The standard oral dose used in clinical practice is 10 mg once daily.

Selegiline in early Parkinson's disease

Systematic review of the monotherapy placebo-controlled trials with selegiline showed that it delays the need for levodopa (odds ratio 0.57; 95% CI 0.48, 0.67; $.P < 0.00001$) and improves UPDRS motor and ADL scores. It also delayed the onset of motor fluctuations (odds ratio 0.75; 95% CI 0.59, 0.95; $.P < 0.02$), but not dyskinesia. This was achieved without any increase in side-effects or withdrawals from treatment.

> Selegiline can be used as initial monotherapy in Parkinson's disease or as adjuvant therapy once motor complications have developed on levodopa

There is no comparative data of selegiline with other monotherapy, such as levodopa or dopamine agonists, so no guidance on which to choose in early PD can be made. Further trials are required in this area.

> Selegiline can cause typical dopaminergic side-effects, but it can also trigger insomnia, nightmares and vivid dreams because of its amphetamine metabolites

Selegiline in later Parkinson's disease

Selegiline adjuvant therapy was evaluated in trials in the mid-1980s. These were mainly small, randomised, controlled trials against placebo and suffered from being short-term and using a variety of different rating scales of motor impairments only. As such, there is no useful data on which to base a systematic review. They seemed to show that selegiline has a significant beneficial effect on motor impairments and that levodopa dose can be reduced, but whether this translates into improvements in quality of life that were worthwhile was not evaluated.

There are no trials comparing adjuvant selegiline therapy with other drug classes, including dopamine agonists and COMT inhibitors. Such trials are required to guide therapy in the future.

Oral fast-melt selegiline

Selegiline has been formulated as a novel oral fast-melt Zydis® preparation which avoids first-pass hepatic metabolism by pre-gastric absorption and so produces fewer amphetamine metabolites than traditional selegiline. A cohort of 163 patients with severe motor fluctuations (> 3 hours 'off' time daily) were randomised to Zydis® selegiline 1.25 mg/day increasing after 6 weeks to 2.5 mg/day for 6 weeks or placebo. The therapeutic gain (treatment effect minus placebo effect) in 'off' time was 5.4% (~0.9 h) on 1.25 mg/day and 9.0% (~1.4 h) on 2.5 mg/day, both improvements being significant compared with placebo. Motor UPDRS scores both 'on' and 'off' improved significantly on Zydis® selegiline compared with placebo and adverse events were acceptable. No trial has compared the Zydis® preparation with traditional selegiline or with any other active adjuvant therapy.

Adverse effects

The adverse event profile of selegiline at any stage of the disease is similar to the other dopamimetic therapies. Thus, nausea, vomiting, postural hypotension, confusion, hallucinations, and insomnia can occur. The latter is often overlooked and can be associated with vivid dreams and nightmares even when taken once daily in the morning.

Rasagiline
Pharmacology

Like selegiline, rasagiline is a propargylamine which is an irreversible inhibitor of MAOB. However, it is not metabolised to amphetamine derivatives like selegiline and so it is potentially free of any alerting side-effects. The licensed oral dose is 1 mg once daily.

Rasagiline in early Parkinson's disease

Two trials have established the efficacy and safety of rasagiline versus placebo. In the larger of these (TEMPO), 404 patients with early PD were randomised to placebo (for 6 months then rasagiline 2 mg/day), rasagiline 1 mg/day or rasagiline 2 mg/day. At 6 months, the licensed dose of 1 mg/day produced a 4.2 unit improvement over placebo in total UPDRS score (95% CI 2.7, 5.7; $P < 0.001$). This trial went on to evaluate whether rasagiline is neuroprotective in PD using a delayed start design (chapter 6).

No trials have compared rasagiline with selegiline in early PD or compared rasagiline with other monotherapy drug classes such as levodopa or dopamine agonists. This work is required to assist in choosing between initial therapies.

Rasagiline can be used as initial monotherapy in PD or as adjuvant therapy once motor complications have developed on levodopa

Rasagiline in later Parkinson's disease

Two large trials and one small one have compared rasagiline with placebo as adjuvant therapy for PD patients with motor complications. In one trial conducted in 472 patients over 26 weeks (PRESTO), the reduction in 'off' time with rasagiline 1 mg/day was 0.94 hours (95% CI 0.51, 1.36; $P < 0.001$) more than with placebo. There were also significant benefits in UPDRS motor and ADL scores, but this did not affect quality of life (PDQUALIF scale). The larger LARGO trial randomised 687 later PD patients to placebo, rasagiline 1 mg/day or entacapone (standard dose) and followed them for 18 weeks. This showed that 'off' time was reduced more than placebo (treatment effect) with both rasagiline (0.78 h; 95% CI 0.39, 1.18; $P < 0.0001$) and entacapone (0.80 h; 95% CI 0.41, 1.20; $P < 0.0001$). UPDRS motor and ADL scores also improved with rasagiline and entacapone to a similar degree.

These trials show that rasagiline is effective, with similar benefits to entacapone. No adjuvant trials have compared rasagiline with selegiline or other adjuvant drug classes such as COMT inhibitors or dopamine agonists. Such trials would be useful to provide data on which to base the choice of drug class in this situation.

Adverse effects

Rasagiline leads to standard dopaminergic adverse effects. There is an increased risk of central nervous system side-effects when SSRIs are given with rasagiline. This is not the case with selegiline, except in the case of escitalopram.

PD MED trial

There is very little trial evidence on whether the addition of a dopamine agonist, a MAOB inhibitor, or a COMT inhibitor is superior in a PD patient with motor complications taking levodopa. This issue is being addressed in the PD MED trial. This study is randomising large numbers of PD patients with motor complications to any dopamine agonist, any MAOB inhibitor or any COMT inhibitor (within statutory regulations) and following their progress with quality of life and health economics outcomes for at least 5 years.

There is insufficient evidence on which to base a decision between adjuvant dopamine agonist, MAOB inhibitor or COMT inhibitor therapy in PD patients who have developed motor complications on levodopa

Amantadine
Brief history

The discovery of the therapeutic value of amantadine in PD was purely fortuitous. During studies in patients with viral illnesses, amantadine was given to a patient with PD who showed a significant improvement in motor function. As a result, a series of small, randomised, placebo-controlled trials were performed with amantadine in the condition in the early 1970s. Following encouraging results, the drug was introduced into clinical practice.

Pharmacology

The mechanism of the central action of amantadine in PD is still uncertain. In the past, actions via dopaminergic and/or cholinergic pathways have been suggested. More recently, it has been found to be a glutamate antagonist.

Clinical use

The original clinical trials with amantadine in PD have undergone Cochrane systematic review, but they suffered from a number of problems, including:

- small sample size
- use of unvalidated clinical rating scales

- inclusion of non-idiopathic cases
- inclusion of patients who had undergone thalamotomy.

However, these studies did demonstrate a beneficial effect on motor impairments. The controlled trials were predominantly short-term (< 12 weeks), but the few long-term controlled and observational studies suggested that tolerance to the effects of amantadine developed with use over 12 weeks. Considering the quality of these trials, such tolerance should be interpreted cautiously.

> Amantadine is now mainly used to reduce dyskinesia in Parkinson's disease patients with later disease

In the past, amantadine was used to delay levodopa therapy in a similar manner to the anticholinergics. This role has now been replaced by the dopamine agonists which may be more effective in treating motor impairments and delaying motor complications, although no direct comparative evidence of this exists. The dose of amantadine should be slowly titrated at weekly intervals to between 100 mg once daily and 100 mg tid.

More recently, amantadine has been examined as an antidyskinetic agent based on the knowledge that it is a glutamate antagonist and that dyskinesia may be mediated through an overactive glutamatergic subthalamopallidal pathway. Early pilot studies have undergone Cochrane systematic review which found encouraging results, but larger and longer trials are now required before amantadine can be firmly recommended to treat dyskinesia.

Adverse effects

Adverse events can be a significant problem with amantadine. Central side-effects such as confusion and hallucinations can occur and peripheral reactions include ankle oedema and livedo reticularis.

β-Adrenergic antagonists

In view of the well-known tremorigenic effect of adrenaline, the first β-adrenergic antagonist to be introduced, pronethalol, in 1963 was tested in a small number of parkinsonian patients with some beneficial results. Unfortunately, pronethalol was withdrawn due to carcinogenesis in mice but was replaced by propranolol. A number of studies examined the anti-tremor action of propranolol in PD in the late 1960s and early 1970s. In common with all of the early studies in the condition, they generally suffered from the drawbacks of:

- a mixed sample of parkinsonism of different aetiologies
- small numbers
- the absence of a control arm
- the use of measures of motor impairment (*e.g.* accelerometry) which had little meaning in terms of ADL and quality of life.

A Cochrane review found only four. randomised, controlled trials comparing β-blocker therapy with placebo in patients with PD. These were double-blind, cross-over studies involving only 72 patients. In view of the paucity of evidence and the poor reporting of the trials, it was impossible to determine whether β-blocker therapy is effective and safe for the treatment of tremor in PD. The high frequency of bradycardia in one trial raised some concerns about the prescription of β-blockers to elderly patients, but the study was too small for the true risk to be evaluated.

> Propranolol can be used to treat postural tremor in Parkinson's disease but the evidence base for its efficacy and safety is poor

Muscarinic antagonists

The muscarinic antagonists or anticholinergics are the oldest of the pharmacotherapies for PD. They first emerged in the late 19th century after Charcot's work with hyoscine (scopolamine). It was not until the mid-20th

Table 9.2
Anticholinergic agents licensed in the UK for the treatment of PD

Generic name	Proprietary name	Therapeutic dose range
Trihexyphenidyl (Benzhexol)	Broflex	2–5 mg tid
Orphenadrine	Disipal, Biorphen	50 mg bd or tid
Procyclidine	Kemadrin, Arpicolin	5–10 mg tid
Benztropine	Cogentin	1–2 mg tid
Biperiden	Akineton	2–4 mg tid

century that relatively selective centrally active muscarinic receptor antagonists were developed with fewer peripheral side-effects. In the absence of alternatives, these agents proliferated and a large number are still available (Table 9.2), although the most commonly used in neurology are trihexyphenidyl (benzhexol) and orphenadrine.

The precise pharmacodynamic action of the muscarinic antagonists is not clear. Generations of medical students have been taught that a 'balance' existed between cholinergic overactivity and dopaminergic underactivity in PD. This concept is too simplistic and the precise relationship between the two neurotransmitter pathways remains uncertain.

A Cochrane review included nine placebo-controlled and active comparator studies of anticholinergics in 221 PD patients, all of which were double-blind cross-over design, with trial durations of 5–20 weeks. As monotherapy or adjunct therapy, anticholinergics were more effective than placebo in improving motor function, but neuropsychiatric and cognitive adverse events occur more frequently on anticholinergics than on placebo and were a more common reason for withdrawal than lack of efficacy. Whether anticholinergics were more effective on tremor than on other outcome measures could not be discerned.

> The anticholinergics can be used to treat severe rest tremor in young PD patients but cognitive impairment and peripheral anticholinergic side effects are extremely common

With the introduction of the more effective levodopa, the use of anticholinergics declined. The recognition in recent years of significant cognitive impairment with these drugs, even in normal volunteers, has led to a further reluctance to use them. They can also precipitate psychotic symptoms including confusion and hallucinations. Peripheral side-effects include nausea, dry mouth, constipation, dizziness, blurred vision, precipitation of closed-angle glaucoma, and urinary retention in prostatic hypertrophy. These are all more common in the elderly in whom these drugs should be avoided.

Further reading

Assal F, Sphar L, Hadengue A, Rubbici-Brandt L, Burkhard P. Tolcapone and fulminant hepatitis. *Lancet* 1998; **352**: 958.

Bonifati V, Meco G. New, selective catechol-O-methyltransferase inhibitors as therapeutic agents in Parkinson's disease. *Pharmacol Ther* 1999; **81**: 1–36.

Clarke CE. Neuroprotection and pharmacotherapy for motor symptoms in Parkinson's disease. *Lancet Neurol* 2004; **3**: 466–75.

Cochrane Library via the Cochrane Collaboration website: <http://www.cochrane.org>.

Crosby N, Deane K, Clarke CE. Beta-blocker therapy for tremor in Parkinson's disease (Cochrane Review). In: *The Cochrane Library*. Chichester, UK: John Wiley, 2003.

Crosby NJ, Deane KHO, Clarke CE. Amantadine for dyskinesia in Parkinson's disease (Cochrane Review). In: *The Cochrane Library*. Chichester, UK: John Wiley, 2003.

Deane K, Spieker S, Clarke CE. Catechol-O-methyl transferase inhibitors for levodopa-induced complications in Parkinson's disease. In: *Cochrane Library*. Chichester, UK: John Wiley; 2004; Issue 4.

Deane K, Spieker S, Clarke CE. Catechol-O-methytransferase inhibitors versus active comparators for levodopa-induced complications in Parkinson's disease. In: *Cochrane Library*. Chichester, UK: John Wiley, 2004; Issue 4.

Ives N, Stowe R, Marro J *et al*. Monoamine oxidase B inhibitor therapy in early Parkinson's disease: a systematic review of randomised controlled trials. *BMJ* 2004; **329**: 593–9.

Katzenschlager R, Sampaio C, Costa J, Lees A. Anticholinergics for symptomatic management of Parkinson's disease (Cochrane Review). In: *The Cochrane Library*. Chichester, UK: John Wiley, 2003.

National Collaborating Centre for Chronic Conditions. Symptomatic pharmacological therapy in Parkinson's disease. In: *Parkinson's disease – National clinical guideline for diagnosis and management in primary and secondary care*. London: Royal College of Physicians, 2006; 59–99.

Parkinson Study Group. A controlled, randomised, delayed-start study of rasagiline in early Parkinson disease. *Arch Neurol* 2004; **61**: 561–6.

Parkinson Study Group. A controlled trial of rasagiline in early Parkinson disease: the TEMPO Study. *Arch Neurol* 2002; **59**: 1937–43.

Parkinson Study Group. A randomized placebo-controlled trial of rasagiline in levodopa-treated patients with Parkinson disease and motor fluctuations: the PRESTO study. *Arch Neurol* 2005; **62**: 241–8.

PD MED website: <http://www.pdmed.bham.ac.uk>.

Rascol O, Brooks D, Melamed E, Oertel W, Poewe W, Stocchi F. Rasagiline as an adjunct to levodopa in Parkinson's disease patients with motor fluctuations (LARGO study): a randomised, double-blind, parallel-group trial. *Lancet* 2005; **365**: 947–54.

10 Non-motor features

Mental health problems
Postural instability and falls
Autonomic disorders
Sleep disorders

Traditionally, most of the emphasis in the management of Parkinson's disease (PD) has been placed on dealing with motor impairments. With the current range of drugs described above, these motor impairments and the motor complications that they give rise to can be managed reasonably well. In recent years, it has been realised that it is now the non-motor disorders in PD that cause the most deterioration in quality of life. Both clinical and research attention is now being turned to these non-motor conditions.

The term 'non-motor' is something of a misnomer. It usually includes all aspects of PD which are not responsive to dopaminergic medication. This includes postural instability and falls which are technically motor disorders.

Mental health problems
Dementia
Definitions

When dementia develops **more than** one year after the onset of the motor features of PD, it is defined as 'Parkinson's disease with dementia (PDD)'. When dementia develops **within** one year of the onset of motor features, it is defined as 'Dementia with Lewy bodies (DLB)'. Since the clinical and pathological features of both of these conditions are similar, it is generally considered that they represent a continuum within the same disorder. Both are referred to collectively here as PD dementias.

Epidemiology

In cross-sectional surveys of PD patients, PD dementias occur in around 40% of patients. However, one longitudinal study showed that 78% of PD patients developed dementia over an 8-year follow-up period. In addition to this high prevalence, dementia has a devastating effect on patients and their carers, with reduction in quality of life and increased economic and social burden. As a consequence, it is now clear that dementia should receive much more clinical attention and should be the focus for further research.

Pathophysiology

In the PD dementias, Lewy bodies are found in cortical and subcortical areas in addition to brainstem nuclei. There is also loss of cholinergic fibres emerging from the brainstem and the nucleus basalis of Meynert.

> Parkinson's disease dementias present with decline in visuospatial abilities, category learning, verbal fluency, set switching, and executive function, rather than the memory loss which occurs in Alzheimer's disease and multiple cerebral infarct dementia

Clinical features

Dementia is the progressive loss of global cognitive function. However, the pattern of cognitive loss is different in the various dementias, although considerable overlap can occur. So, in Alzheimer's disease and multiple cerebral infarct dementia, there is a predominant amnestic syndrome (*i.e.* memory loss). In contrast, in the PD dementias, there is impairment in visuospatial abilities, category learning, verbal fluency, set switching, and executive function (*i.e.* working memory, mental flexibility and the ability to initiate and suppress responses).

The clinical features of PD dementias can also be differentiated by additional features:

- visual hallucinations
- fluctuating course, often with lucid intervals
- extrapyramidal features suggesting PD.

Helpful features in the diagnosis of Parkinson's disease dementias are fluctuations in cognition, with 'good days and bad days', visual hallucinations and the motor features of Parkinson's disease

Management

PD dementias evolve over several years, often beginning with subtle features such as nightmares, nocturnal confusion and daytime somnolence. It is only when more frank problems with activities of daily living develop that a formal diagnosis is made. In terms of management, this gradual evolution usually means that the patient initially suffers from psychotic features which require the management strategy outlined in the next section.

The cholinesterase inhibitors rivastigmine, donepezil, and galantamine have been developed to treat the cognitive impairments in Alzheimer's disease. Considerable debate surrounds their efficacy in this condition: whilst short-term pharmaceutical industry trials have shown clear benefits, the AD2000 trial found no effect on institutionalisation or mortality over a mean of 3 years' follow-up. There was an initial reluctance to evaluate cholinesterase inhibitors in PD dementias because of the relative cholinergic excess in the striatum which contributes to motor dysfunction and leads to the effectiveness of anticholinergics in the condition. However, the evidence from randomised, placebo-controlled trials of cholinesterase inhibitors in both PDD and DLB show that they are effective and safe and that they do not cause any significant decline in motor function. Cholinesterase inhibitors are effective in treating not only the cognitive decline but the psychotic features of

the condition. Not all patients respond and side-effects can be prohibitive, so regular review is required. At present, only rivastigmine has a product licence in the UK, but a large trial with donepezil is about to be reported.

Cholinesterase inhibitors can reduce psychotic features and improve cognition in some patients with Parkinson's disease dementias

Whilst the cholinesterase inhibitors provide limited symptomatic relief for some patients with PD dementias, definitive neuroprotective therapy for PD is required to slow its progression so that patients do not develop dementia in the first place.

Psychosis

Clinical features

Psychosis in PD often begins with mild features including vivid dreams, illusions (distortion of sensory perceptions), and non-frightening visual hallucinations (strong perception of an event or object when no such situation is present) of animals or people. Patients will often tolerate these mild symptoms. However, eventually, more severe psychotic symptoms develop with paranoid delusions and upsetting visual hallucinations.

Psychotic symptoms are often the first sign of dementia in Parkinson's disease

Pathophysiology

Psychosis is often caused by underlying PD dementia or the patient's medication. Even relatively young patients can develop psychosis when they first start medication, more commonly with a dopamine agonist. Quite why they are so sensitive is not known, although such patients should be watched carefully for the onset of dementia. When psychosis develops in later disease, without any recent change in medication, it is usually the harbinger of dementia.

The pathophysiology of psychosis is not fully understood. Whilst the dopaminergic pathways to the limbic system and cortex may be implicated, other degenerate catecholaminergic pathways may be involved, along with the cholinergic deficiency which is seen in PD dementias.

> Older, 'typical' antipsychotics, such as haloperidol, should never be used in Parkinson's disease psychosis as they are dopamine antagonists which precipitate severe and prolonged motor decline

Management

The management of psychosis in PD is outlined in Table 10.1. The first step in the management of psychosis is to decide with the patient and carer whether the symptoms are sufficiently distressing to require intervention. Many patients are reasonably happy to continue with occasional visual hallucinations of people sitting next to them or animals, knowing they are not real. In this situation, no change in treatment may be necessary.

Any precipitating medical condition, such as infection or dehydration, must be treated.

The next step is to withdraw any recently commenced antiparkinsonian medication which may be the precipitant. Thereafter, minor agents such as anticholinergics, amantadine, and selegiline should be withdrawn. This may

Table 10.1
Management of psychosis in Parkinson's disease

- Treat any precipitating medical condition (e.g. infection or dehydration)
- Slowly reduce then withdraw anticholinergics, selegiline, amantadine, and dopamine agonists – 'last one in, first one out' rule
- If absolutely necessary, reduce levodopa slowly and accept deteriorating mobility
- Consider adding an atypical antipsychotic (e.g. clozapine)
- Consider adding a cholinesterase inhibitor
- Prevent complications of immobility (e.g. DVT prophylaxis)

only have a small impact on the patient's motor function. Then dopamine agonists and levodopa should be reduced cautiously accepting a significant decline in mobility. This can be the point at which more intensive carer and community support is required and, occasionally, residential home admission.

An alternative approach at any point in the above scheme is to consider adding an antipsychotic agent. The older generation antipsychotics (e.g. haloperidol) block dopaminergic transmission in motor pathways, so patient's motor function deteriorates. This led to the search for modern antipsychotics which do not cause deterioration in motor function. A number of small trials have shown that the atypical neuroleptic clozapine can reduce psychotic symptoms. However, neutropenia occurs in 1–2% of patients, so detailed monitoring is required. Clozapine has a product licence for use in PD psychosis in the UK and blood monitoring and prescription co-ordination can be arranged.

Studies with risperidone and olanzapine in PD psychosis have shown that motor function deteriorates with these agents. The early work with quetiapine was more hopeful, but more recent controlled studies have been negative.

The 5-HT$_3$ receptor antagonist ondansetron is used as an anti-emetic in oncology. Some small trials have suggested that it may be useful in parkinsonian psychosis without interfering with motor function. Further work is required before this expensive drug can be recommended.

The beneficial effects of the cholinesterase inhibitors on psychotic symptoms in PD dementias raises the possibility that these may become the most effective treatment for psychosis in PD without frank dementia.

Depression

Epidemiology

Depression is a major clinical problem in patients with PD. The prevalence of depression in PD has varied widely in observational studies between 4% and 90% depending on the criteria used for diagnosis and whether studies were community- or hospital-based. In a meta-analysis of 26 studies in 1992, the mean prevalence of depression was calculated to be 40%. In a more recent Norwegian community-based study, depression was found in 26% of patients. In a community-based study in North Wales, depression was found in 64% of patients with PD referred to a geriatric service and in 34% of their carers.

> Depression affects around 40% of patients with PD and leads to significant reduction in quality of life

The impact of depression on the lives of patients with PD has further been underlined in recent years by quality-of-life studies. For example, a Norwegian community-based study examined quality of life in 233 patients with PD using the Nottingham Health Profile. It revealed that 54% of the reduction in quality of life could be explained by depression, sleep problems, low Schwab and England score (disease-specific ADL scale), low UPDRS motor score, and levodopa dose. Similarly, the Global Parkinson's Disease Survey examined quality of life using the PDQ 39 questionnaire in over 1000 PD patients in six countries. This revealed that more than 40% of the reduction in quality of life was explained by depression compared with 17% for Hoehn and Yahr stage and medication.

The current practice of many clinicians when assessing a patient with PD in the clinic is to concentrate on motor impairments and the patient's response to therapy. The high prevalence of depression and these quality-of-life data suggest that this attitude to clinic assessment is inadequate and that we must develop ways of routinely looking for depression in all PD patients.

> Clinicians and Parkinson's Disease Nurse Specialists should have a low index of suspicion for depression in Parkinson's disease

The prevalence of depression in PD is greater than occurs in other chronic disorders with similar levels of disability. This, combined with the occurrence of depression before the onset of motor disability and the lack of a correlation between its severity and motor disability, suggests that a significant proportion of depression in PD is endogenous and perhaps part of the disease process rather than a reaction to the disability.

Pathophysiology

The neural mechanism of depression in PD is unknown. It is tempting to suggest that dopamine depletion is the cause, since this is the underlying pathology of PD: reserpine depletes dopamine from storage vesicles and so causes depression. Depression can develop during PD patients' 'off' periods. However, treatment to reverse dopamine deficiency, such as levodopa, does not reverse depression, in spite of increasing mesolimbic dopamine. Noradrenaline and 5-hydroxytryptophan are also depleted in PD and may play a part in the genesis of depression.

Management

The wide spectrum of depression in PD ranges between very mild depressive symptoms, which may not require any treatment, through to severe depression requiring formal psychiatric evaluation, pharmacotherapy and even electroconvulsive therapy (ECT).

A Cochrane review and two subsequent randomised, controlled trials have addressed the effectiveness of antidepressant therapies in PD versus placebo or active comparator. No controlled trials were found on ECT or cognitive behavioural therapy. The Cochrane review failed to find any significant benefit of nortriptyline (tricyclic class antidepressant) over placebo, citalopram (selective serotonin re-uptake inhibitor [SSRI] class) over placebo or fluvoxamine (SSRI class) over amitriptyline (tricyclic class). A subsequent trial comparing sertraline (SSRI class) and placebo found no significant difference in depression ratings. The final trial found that both transcranial magnetic stimulation and fluoxetine (SSRI class) improved depression, but there were no significant differences between them. All of these trials had methodological limitations including small sample sizes (range, 22–47) and short duration (16–52 weeks).

In the treatment of depression in PD, it is clear that there is insufficient evidence on the efficacy and safety of all classes of antidepressant pharmacotherapy, cognitive behavioural therapy and ECT. There is an urgent need for further research to establish effective and safe treatments for depression in PD.

> Clinical trials of all types of antidepressant therapies in Parkinson's disease have been poor and inconclusive, so no guidance can be given for clinical practice

Postural instability and falls

Postural instability and falls usually occur late in the course of PD. They are difficult to treat and respond poorly to increases in antiparkinsonian medication. Falls frequently lead to fractures which can be life-threatening but, at least, reduce quality of life and increase the costs of care.

> Falls early in the course of a parkinsonian syndrome suggest progressive supranuclear palsy or multiple cerebral infarction

Instability can be demonstrated by the 'pull test' in which the patient stands with feet slightly apart and, after a warning from the examiner, is pulled sharply backwards at the shoulders. If the patient falls uncontrollably backwards into the examiner's hands, the test is positive.

Treatment should follow the NICE guidelines on falls management and the National Service Framework for the Elderly. This will usually involve a multidisciplinary assessment of the patient, preferably within their own home, by

an experienced team of physiotherapists and occupational therapists, along with a full medical review. Strategies such as walking aids (e.g. sticks, frames) may be required and certain flooring surfaces such as thick pile carpet may have to be removed.

> Falls' management requires a multidisciplinary assessment of the Parkinson's disease patient, preferably in their home

Ultimately, in spite of the best medical and allied health professional efforts, recurrent falls can be the final straw which leads to residential care placement.

Autonomic disorders
Constipation

Constipation is extremely common, if not universal, in PD. It can even occur before the onset of the motor disorder. It is probably caused by direct involvement of the myenteric plexus in the pathology of the condition as Lewy bodies are found in the gut wall. Management should follow a pragmatic policy of increased fluids, fruit and fibre, leading on to the use of laxatives individually then in combination depending on the patient's response.

> Constipation should initially be treated with increased fluids, fruit, and fibre. If therapeutic trials of several laxatives used on their own fail, a combination of agents from different drug classes should be used together

Bladder dysfunction

Severe urinary problems, particularly early in the course of PD, raise the prospect of an alternative diagnosis, such as multiple system atrophy, or concurrent conditions such as prostatism. The physical limitations of the patient's motor disabilities must also be considered: they may not be able to get to the toilet in time.

Early bladder disturbance suggests an alternative diagnosis such as MSA or another problem such as prostatism

However, a significant proportion of PD patients develop mild-to-moderate detrusor hyper-reflexia due to central abnormalities in the pontine micturition centre. These do respond to peripheral antimuscarinic agents, such as oxybutynin and tolterodine, which are generally well tolerated.

Moderate detrusor hyper-reflexia can be controlled with oxybutynin or tolterodine

Orthostatic hypotension

Orthostatic hypotension (OH) occurs in 48% of patients with PD, but is asymptomatic in a large proportion of these cases. It is defined as a drop in systolic blood pressure after standing greater than or equal to 20 mmHg or to a level less than 90 mmHg. OH occurs in PD because of Lewy body degeneration in the hypothalamus, brainstem and peripheral nervous system. Symptoms of OH include fatigue, pre-syncope, syncope, and falls.

The initial management of OH includes reduction in antihypertensive medication, reduction or change in anti-parkinsonian drugs, increase dietary salt and fluid intake, eating small frequent meals, avoiding alcohol, and elevation head of bed by 30–40°. If necessary, the salt-retaining steroid fludrocortisone can be used. The direct-acting sympathomimetic midodrine is rarely required.

Sleep disorders

Sleep disturbance occurs in nearly all patients with PD. Patients should be asked about sleep problems regularly and, if present, a thorough sleep history should be taken (Table 10.2).

The specific sleep disorders restless legs' syndrome (RLS) and rapid eye movement (REM) sleep behaviour disorder (RBD) are considered in chapter 4.

Table 10.2
Points to include in a sleep history

- Details of the three phases of sleep – initiation, maintenance and awakening
- Presence of depression
- Presence of periodic leg movements in sleep
- Presence of vivid dreams and/or hallucinations
- Presence of restless legs' syndrome
- Presence of acting out of dreams (RBD)
- Presence of daytime hypersomnolence
- Drug history (e.g. selegiline causing nightmares)

Daytime hypersomnolence is very common in PD and is often due to dopaminergic medication. There have been recent reports of sudden onset of sleep in patients with PD which were originally attributed to dopamine agonists. However, it is now clear that this can occur with levodopa. Often, daytime sleepiness is caused by poor sleep at night, so-called inversion of the sleep–wake cycle. Hypersomnolence can also be caused by dementia due to poor attention span.

The management of sleep disturbance relies on good sleep hygiene to avoid inverting the sleep–wake cycle: ensuring regular bedtimes and not allowing naps during the day. Short-acting benzodiazepines such as temazepam can be useful. Improved treatment of daytime motor problems seems to help nocturnal difficulties. The evidence base for using modafinil to improve alertness during the day is poor, but this agent does have a product licence for use in the UK for this indication.

Nocturnal akinesia is a common problem as most PD patients take their last antiparkinsonian medication with their evening meal, so they are 'off' overnight. This is manifest as difficulty in turning over in bed and difficulty in getting to the toilet. Nocturnal akinesia can be helped with a dose of modified-release levodopa last thing at night and by aids from an occupational therapist (e.g. silk sheets).

Further reading

Aarsland D, Andersen K, Larsen JP *et al*. Prevalence and characteristics of dementia in Parkinson disease: an 8-year prospective study. *Arch Neurol* 2003; **60**: 387–92.

Barone P, Amboni M, Vitale C *et al*. Treatment of nocturnal disturbances and excessive daytime sleepiness in Parkinson's disease. *Neurology* 2004; **63 (Suppl 3)**: S35–8.

Brown RG, MacCarthy B. Psychiatric morbidity in patients with Parkinson's disease. *Psychol Med* 1990; **20**: 77–87.

Chaudhuri KR, Forbes A, Grosset DG *et al*. Diagnosing restless legs syndrome (RLS) in primary care. *Curr Med Res Opin* 2004; **20**: 1785–95.

Cummings JL. Depression and Parkinson's disease: a review. *Am J Psychiatry* 1992; **4**: 443–54.

Emre M, Aarsland D, Albanese A *et al*. Rivastigmine for dementia associated with Parkinson's disease. *N Engl J Med* 2004; **351**: 2509–18.

Findley L, Peto V, Pugner K, Holmes J, Baker M, MacMahon DG. The impact of Parkinson's disease on quality of life: results of a research survey in the UK. *Mov Disord* 2000; **15 (Suppl 3)**: 179.

Fregni F, Santos CM, Myczkowski ML *et al*. Repetitive transcranial magnetic stimulation is as effective as fluoxetine in the treatment of depression in patients with Parkinson's disease. *J Neurol Neurosurg Psychiatry* 2004; **75**: 1171–4.

Frucht S, Rogers JD, Greene PE *et al*. Falling asleep at the wheel: motor vehicle mishaps in persons taking pramipexole and ropinirole. *Neurology* 1999; **52**: 1908–10.

Karlsen KH, Larsen JP, Tandberg E, Maeland JG. Influence of clinical and demographic variables on quality of life in patients with Parkinson's disease. *J Neurol Neurosurg Psychiatry* 1999; **66**: 431–5.

Leentjens AF, Vreeling FW, Luijckx GJ *et al*. SSRIs in the treatment of depression in Parkinson's disease. *Int J Geriatr Psychiatry* 2003; **18**: 552–4.

Lees AJ, Blackburn NA, Campbell VL. The night-time problems of Parkinson's disease. *Clin Neuropharmacol* 1988; **11**: 512–9.

McKeith I, Del Ser T, Spano P *et al*. Efficacy of rivastigmine in dementia with Lewy bodies: a randomised, double-blind, placebo-controlled international study. *Lancet* 2000; **356**: 2031–6.

Meara J, Mitchelmore E, Hobson P. Use of the GDS-15 geriatric depression scale as a screening instrument for depressive symptomatology in patients with Parkinson's disease and their carers in the community. *Age Ageing* 1999; **28**: 35–8.

National Collaborating Centre for Chronic Conditions. Non-motor features of Parkinson's disease. In: *Parkinson's disease – National clinical guideline for diagnosis and management in primary and secondary care*. London: Royal College of Physicians, 2006; 113–34.

NICE Clinical Guideline no. 21. *Falls: assessment and prevention of falls in older people*. 2004. Available from <www.nice.org.uk>.

Shabnam G, Chung TH, Deane KHO *et al*. Therapies for depression in Parkinson's disease (Cochrane Review). *Cochrane Database of Systematic Reviews*. 2003; 2: CD003465.

Tandberg E, Larsen JP, Aarsland D, Cummings JL. The occurrence of depression in Parkinson's disease. A community-based study. *Arch Neurol* 1996; **53**: 175–9.

11 Surgical management

Functional neurosurgery
Intracerebral grafting
Other forms of surgery

Functional neurosurgery

Brief history

With the lack of adequate therapy for Parkinson's disease (PD) and the evolution of safe neurosurgery, various surgical approaches to the condition were attempted in the 1930s and 1940s. Lesions were placed in the corticospinal pathway in the spinal cord, the dentate nucleus of the cerebellum, and the premotor cortex with little beneficial effect and considerable morbidity and mortality.

In 1952, Cooper ligated the anterior choroidal artery by accident in a patient with PD whilst attempting another operation. The beneficial effects of this procedure led to further operations with variable results, but it did encourage others to explore lesioning of the outflow pathways from the globus pallidus. The mixed success of such procedures was probably due to poor localisation techniques. This improved with the availability of accurate three-dimensional targeting using stereotaxis, which had originally been introduced by Spiegel and Wycis in 1946. The breakthrough came in 1960 when Leksell's group found that lesions placed in the posteroventral portion of the medial segment of the globus pallidus produced significant benefits in parkinsonian symptoms.

The dramatic success of levodopa in the 1960s then quashed further surgical development. However, the poor effects of levodopa on tremor left the way clear for lesioning of the ventralis intermedius (VIM) nucleus of the thalamus (thalamotomy) which was found to be more effective for tremor than the other features of the condition. It was only in the early 1990s that Laitinen returned to posteroventral pallidotomy for more severe disease associated with motor complications which were unresponsive to pharmacotherapy. However, thalamotomy and pallidotomy are destructive procedures with a relatively high morbidity.

Significant strides in the understanding of the neural mechanisms of movement disorders were made in the 1990s, largely thanks to work in animal models such as the MPTP model of PD (chapters 2 and 3). Technical improvements in functional neurosurgery occurred at the same time, including the advent of MRI stereotaxis. This led to the development of subthalamic (STN) deep-brain stimulation (DBS) for unresponsive motor complications in PD. The dramatic success of this procedure led to an explosion in the interest in functional neurosurgery for intractable motor complications in PD.

However, the incidence of these severe motor complications is falling as less reliance is placed on high-dose levodopa therapy, so it is likely that STN-DBS will be required less frequently in the future. Attention now must turn to neurorestorative surgical approaches which increase the number of dopaminergic neurones, whether this is by implantation of dopamine producing tissue or the infusion of nerve growth factors.

> Bilateral subthalamic deep brain stimulation is appropriate for a small number of Parkinson's disease patients with severe motor complications which cannot be managed by medical therapy

Rationale

The functional anatomy of the basal ganglia was outlined in chapter 3 and is reprised in Figure 11.1. In essence, movement is controlled by a pathway which passes from the premotor cortex through the striatum (putamen and caudate) and globus pallidus to the thalamus and then back to the supplementary motor cortex. Activity in this loop is modulated by the substantia nigra, which acts like a motor car accelerator, and the STN, which acts like a brake. In PD, the nigra is defective, so the accelerator fails to work and the patient slows down. Following a stroke involving the STN, the brake is lost and the patient speeds up developing involuntary movements in the contralateral limbs (hemiballismus/hemichorea syndrome).

On the assumption that the 'accelerator' and 'brake' pathways work separately in a constant equilibrium (unlike a motor vehicle), a logical approach to the treatment of PD (in which the 'accelerator' is lost) is to switch off the 'brake'. This means reducing over-activity in the glutamatergic pathway from the STN to the medial segment of the globus pallidus (GPM)

and/or reducing the over-activity in the gabaminergic pathway from the GPM to the thalamus.

Reducing the activity of a pathway can be achieved by either lesioning it or over-stimulating it so that it switches off physiologically (depolarisation blockade). Lesioning is most commonly performed by stereotactic thermocoagulation in which an electrode is accurately targeted through a burr hole in the skull to the site in question using MRI, an electric current is then passed through the electrode tip which heats up to a set temperature for a carefully judged period. Deep brain stimulation (DBS) is achieved using similar technology to a cardiac pacemaker. An electrode is placed in the target using MRI stereotaxy (Fig. 11.2), along with neurophysiological monitoring of brain activity as the electrode descends through the brain to the target. The electrode is then connected via

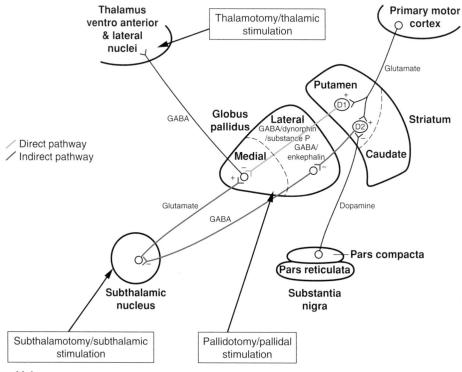

Figure 11.1
Sites of action of functional neurosurgical techniques.

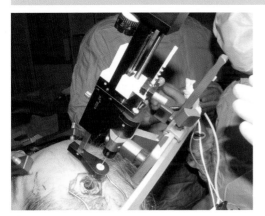

Figure 11.2
Surgical location of an electrode for STN deep brain stimulation in PD.
Courtesy of Mrs R Mitchell.

wiring tunnelled under the skin to a pulse generator ('pacing' box) placed under the anterior chest wall skin (Fig. 11.3). The latter can then be programmed through the intact skin with an external probe connected to a computer (Fig. 11.4). The location of the electrodes can be checked during the operation with a standard radiograph (Fig. 11.5) and after the operation by MRI (Fig. 11.6).

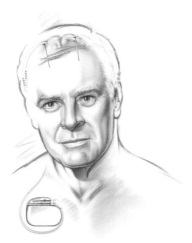

Figure 11.3
Schematic drawing of bilateral STN deep brain stimulation system in PD.
Courtesy of Medtronic.

Bilateral subthalamic deep brain stimulation

The relatively high morbidity and mortality of lesioning operations such as thalamotomy and pallidotomy have led to them being abandoned in favour of bilateral STN-DBS. In general, biologically fit and non-demented patients with PD whose involuntary movements or 'off' periods cannot be controlled with changes in medical therapy are suitable for STN-DBS. The procedure is particularly good at reducing 'off' time and 'off' time disability, so that medication can be reduced thereby reducing dyskinesia.

Subthalamic deep-brain stimulation reduces 'off' time and 'off' time disability so that medication can be reduced thereby reducing dyskinesia

In spite of the wide-spread acceptance of STN-DBS, the evidence base for its efficacy and safety leaves much to be desired. The 'evolution' of the procedure occurred through a large number of case series with initially no randomised, controlled trials against pre-existing best medical therapy or chronic apomorphine infusions. These non-controlled trials have recently been reviewed. This showed that STB-DBS reduced 'off' period UPDRS motor (27%) and ADL scores (13%), reduced levodopa dose equivalents (56%),

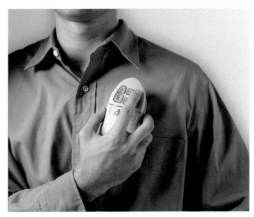

Figure 11.4
Patient control for STN deep brain stimulation system in PD.
Courtesy of Medtronic.

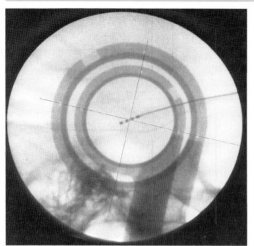

Figure 11.5
Radiograph taken during surgery to check location of the quadripolar electrode for STN deep brain stimulation in PD.
Courtesy of Mrs R Mitchell.

reduced dyskinesia (69%; UPDRS scores 32–35), and improved quality of life (35%; PDQ 39). However, this was at the expense of 3.9% of patients developing intracranial haemorrhage related to surgery. Psychiatric side-effects, such as depression, suicide, psychosis and hallucinations, were common. Technical problems with lead fracture, infection and battery replacement also occurred. The drawbacks of STN-DBS include its substantial cost. It has been estimated using UK 2002 prices that the procedure costs

£32,526 per PD patient over 5 years; 70% of these costs are attributable to the initial costs of the equipment and its replacement costs in the future. An American study using 2000 prices estimated the incremental cost effectiveness ratio (ICER) of STN-DBS in PD to be around $49,000 (~£27,000; 2006 conversion) per QALY. A similar study using UK 1998 prices performed as part of the recent NICE guidelines process suggested an ICER of £19,500 per QALY.

> In spite of the wide-spread acceptance of subthalamic deep-brain stimulation, further information is required on its long-term cost-benefits and side-effects

The non-controlled case series published to date with STN-DBS have been relatively small (range, 10–96 patients) and short-term (mean follow-up, 15 months). Also, the absence of randomisation can lead to significant bias from patient selection factors. Future trials need to place more emphasis on patient-rated quality of life and to assess the cost-benefits of the procedure. The long-term safety of STN-DBS is also of some concern. Cases of severe depression leading to suicide are unusual in PD, but have been recorded after STN-DBS.

In an attempt to resolve these outstanding issues, two randomised trials of STN-DBS versus

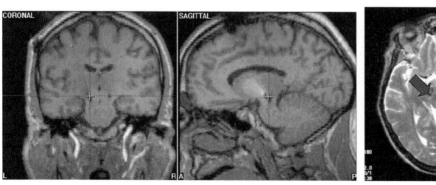

Figure 11.6
Postoperative MRI to check location of the electrodes for STN deep brain stimulation in PD.
Courtesy of Mrs R Mitchell.

best medical therapy/delayed surgery are underway. A German trial in 156 patients has shown significant improvements in quality of life (PDQ 39) at 6 months in the surgery group. A larger 10-year trial is on-going in the UK at present (PD SURG) funded by the Medical Research Council (MRC) and the Parkinson's Disease Society.

In spite of these uncertainties, a NICE Intervention Procedure Guidance and the recent NICE PD guidelines are supportive of the procedure, with the caveat that PD SURG is on-going and that patients should be encouraged to join the trial.

Bilateral globus pallidus deep brain stimulation

Switching off the overactive gabaminergic output of the medial segment of the globus pallidus to the thalamus with DBS is an alternative to STN-DBS. The very few, small, short-term case-series of this procedure are insufficient to make any definitive comments on its efficacy and safety, so the STN continues to be the most common target for functional neurosurgery for PD.

Intracerebral grafting

The possibility of transplanting embryonic dopaminergic neurones into the striatum to relieve the symptoms of PD was first explored in the early 1980s by Bjorklund and Dunnett in the 6-hydroxydopamine rat model of the condition. They showed that the implanted cells survived and produced synaptic contacts with the host which allowed some functional recovery.

The earliest trial of human fetal grafts in four patients with PD by Lindvall's team in Sweden was not encouraging, probably because of poor graft survival, as evidenced by low ^{18}F-fluorodopa uptake shown on PET imaging. In a more recent cohort of patients, the Swedish group has had more success with mean increases in ^{18}F-fluorodopa uptake of 68%, 12 months after surgery. This was

accompanied by improvements in motor impairments and, in one case, the ability to withdraw levodopa completely. In the single post-mortem on a patient 18 months after such a graft, 10% of the putamen was found to be re-innervated.

In view of these encouraging results, two North American trials of fetal implantation were performed. Rather controversially, but scientifically appropriate, both trials included a sham surgery control arm in which patients had a burr hole but no graft; these control patients went on to receive grafts at the end of the trial. Both trials showed that the grafts led to small improvement in motor function and ADL in some patients, along with increases in ^{18}F-fluorodopa uptake shown on PET. However, a prohibitive amount of dyskinesia and dystonia, especially in 'off' periods, developed in grafted patients which had not been seen in the Swedish studies. These complications were so severe that pallidotomy was necessary in some patients.

> Novel treatment approaches to Parkinson's disease which include implanting new dopamine producing cells may suffer from unregulated transmitter release and thus severe 'off' period dyskinesia and dystonia

The inability to control the over production of dopamine by these fetal grafts has halted further development of this technique. The need for midbrain cells from four aborted human fetuses for each putamen graft also presented considerable ethical and practical problems. This may be overcome by using an alternative supply of dopamine-producing cells.

Experiments in rats have shown that it is possible to grow host fibroblast cells taken from skin biopsies in tissue culture, transfect them with the gene for tyrosine hydroxylase, then transplant colonies of cells manufacturing levodopa into the 6-hydroxydopamine-treated host which generate significant functional recovery.

A clinical trial has also been done with human retinal pigment epithelial cells which produce dopamine and can be attached to gelatin microcarriers. In six patients, these grafts improved 'off' period UPDRS motor scores by 48% at 12 months and no 'off' period dyskinesias were seen. A further trial with this type of graft is currently underway.

Attention is now focusing on the production of dopamine-producing cell lines from stem cells for grafting in PD. It will probably take around 10–20 years to achieve such stable cell lines, to perform trials of their implantation in animal models and then patients, and finally to overcome the very likely problems of over stimulation by regulating dopamine release in some way.

Other forms of surgery

An alternative way to restore dopaminergic innervation to the striatum is to stimulate the remaining dopaminergic neurones to produce more fibres and thus more dopamine. This could potentially be achieved by administering a nerve growth factor.

This approach has been used in PD using recombinant glial cell line-derived neurotrophic factor (GDNF). Initial trials infusing GDNF into the ventricles were unsuccessful. GDNF was then infused directly into the putamen in five PD patients with quite dramatic improvements in 'off' period UPDRS motor and ADL scores and ^{18}F-fluorodopa uptake shown on PET. However, small, uncontrolled trials tend to produce such dramatic results which cannot be confirmed in larger controlled studies. A randomised, placebo-controlled trial of GDNF infusion into the putamen of 34 PD patients failed to show a predetermined level of benefit at 6 months, so the trial was stopped. This failure may have been due to technical problems with the way the infusions were administered, but additional problems included neutralising antibodies to the GDNF preparation in three patients and the subsequent finding of cerebellar damage in non-human primates given GDNF.

Further reading

Freed CR, Greene PE, Breeze RE et al. Transplantation of embryonic dopamine neurons for severe Parkinson's disease. N Engl J Med 2001; **344**: 710–9.

Gill SS, Patel NK, Hotton GR et al. Direct brain infusion of glial cell line-derived neurotrophic factor in Parkinson's disease. Nat Med 2003; **9**: 589–95.

Kleiner-Fisman G, Herzog J, Fisman DN et al. Subthalamic nucleus deep brain stimulation: summary and meta-analysis of outcomes. Mov Disord 2006; **21 (Suppl 14)**: S290–304.

Kordower JH, Freeman TB, Snow BJ et al. Neuropathological evidence of graft survival and striatal reinnervation after the transplantation of fetal mesencephalic tissue in a patient with Parkinson's disease. N Engl J Med 1995; **332**: 1118–24.

Lang AE, Gill SS, Patel NK et al. Randomised controlled trial of intraputaminal glial cell line-derived neurotrophic factor in Parkinson's disease. Ann Neurol 2006; **59**: 459–66.

Lindvall O, Rechncrona S, Brundin P et al. Human fetal dopamine neurones grafted into the striatum in two patients with Parkinson's disease. Arch Neurol 1989; **46**: 615–31.

McIntosh E, Gray A, Aziz T. Estimating the costs of surgical innovations: the case of subthalamic nucleus stimulation in the treatment of advanced Parkinson's disease. Mov Disord 2003; **18**: 993–9.

National Collaborating Centre for Chronic Conditions. Surgery for Parkinson's disease. In: Parkinson's disease – National clinical guideline for diagnosis and management in primary and secondary care. London: Royal College of Physicians, 2006; 101–12.

National Institute for Health and Clinical Excellence. Intervention Procedure Guidance 19: Deep brain stimulation for Parkinson's disease. London: NICE, 2003.

Olanow CW, Goetz CG, Kordower JH et al. A double-blind controlled trial of bilateral fetal nigral transplantation in Parkinson's disease. Ann Neurol 2003; **54**: 403–14.

PD SURG website: <http://www.pdsurg.bham.ac.uk>.

Shimohama S, Fisher LJ, Gage FH. Intracerebral grafting of genetically modified cells. Adv Neurol 1993; **60**: 744–8.

Stover NP, Bakay RAE, Subramanian T et al. Intrastriatal implantation of human retinal pigment epithelial cells attached to microcarriers in advanced Parkinson's disease. Arch Neurol 2005; **62**: 1833–7.

Stowe R, Wheatley K, Clarke CE et al. Surgery for Parkinson's disease: lack of reliable clinical trial evidence. J Neurol Neurosurg Psychiatry 2003; **74**: 519–21.

Tomaszewski K, Holloway RG. Deep brain stimulation in the treatment of Parkinson's disease: a cost effectiveness analysis. Neurology 2001; **57**: 663–71.

12 Other interventions

Allied health professionals
Parkinson's Disease Nurse Specialists

Despite optimal medical and occasionally surgical therapy, patients with Parkinson's disease (PD) suffer increasing disability and handicap due to the disease. This leads to reduced quality of life for both the patient and his or her carer, and increased costs for the family and the country as a whole. Earlier chapters have discussed the need for further work on issues such as depression and dementia particularly when motor function has been treated as far as possible. However, there is a potential for improving handicap and quality of life, and possibly reducing costs, using alternative interventions provided by allied health professionals (AHPs) and Parkinson's Disease Nurse Specialists (PDNSs).

Allied health professionals

Rehabilitation should be provided by a multidisciplinary team (Fig. 12.1). Many secondary care facilities treating PD in the UK have multidisciplinary teams, particularly departments of geriatric medicine. However, this is not universal and most neurologists struggle to refer their patients for such services as out-patients. In one survey of 72 consecutive PD patients attending a neurology clinic, only 29% had seen a physiotherapist, 18% an occupational therapist, and 15% a speech and language therapist. This low referral rate reflects multiple issues, including:

- the paucity of such therapy services in the UK which are already overburdened
- a perceived lack of data on the efficacy and effectiveness of paramedical therapies in PD.

These two major issues are linked. Without adequate information on the value of paramedical therapies in PD, healthcare purchasers will not invest in such services.

Physiotherapy

The purpose of physiotherapy in PD is to maximise functional ability and minimise secondary complications through movement rehabilitation within a context of education and support for the whole person. Many physiotherapy methods have been advocated in PD, including:

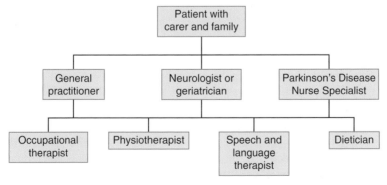

Figure 12.1
The multidisciplinary team in PD.

- proprioceptive neuromuscular facilitation – active muscle contractions, muscle stretch, patterns of movement, resistance, and verbal and visual cues mainly aimed at reducing rigidity
- Bobath – reducing abnormal muscle tone and posture using inhibiting techniques and postures, and facilitation of correct movement through handling by the therapist
- conductive education – reduction of dependency on aids and facilitation of participation in society
- *ad hoc* combinations of the above and other techniques
- miscellaneous methods such as karate, spinal flexibility exercises and balance training.

The Cochrane systematic review of any physiotherapy technique versus a placebo or sham intervention (often no intervention) located only 11 trials with 280 patients. Eight trials did not have adequate placebo treatments, all used a small number of patients, and the method of randomisation and concealment of allocation was good in only four trials. These methodological problems could potentially lead to bias from a number of sources. Although 10 trials claimed a positive effect from physiotherapy, few outcomes measured were statistically significant. Walking velocity was measured in four studies and increased significantly in two. However, there was significant heterogeneity in both trial design and the results due to the large positive effect of one in-patient trial, the remaining physiotherapy regimens being carried out in out-patient departments or at home. Stride length was the only other outcome measured in more than one trial; it significantly improved by 22% (two trials). Five other outcomes improved significantly in individual studies, but eight other outcomes did not.

The authors of the review concluded that, in view of the relatively small number of patients examined, the methodological flaws in most of the studies and the high likelihood of

publication bias (as negative trials tend not to get published), there was insufficient evidence to support or refute the efficacy of physiotherapy in PD. They suggested that large, well-designed, placebo-controlled, randomised, control trials are needed to demonstrate the efficacy and effectiveness of physiotherapy in PD, with particular emphasis on the use of outcome measures with relevance to patients, carers, physicians and physiotherapists, and monitoring these for at least 6 months to determine the duration of any carryover effect.

The same group has performed the Cochrane review of one type of physiotherapy versus another. This found seven trials in 142 patients but, since there is no established 'gold standard' form of therapy against which to compare a novel type, these studies examined many varied types of therapy which could not be quantitatively summated. The individual studies were too small to demonstrate the superiority of one form of therapy over another, particularly considering their methodological flaws and possibility of publication bias.

It must be emphasised that the absence of evidence for a positive effect of physiotherapy in PD does not imply the absence of an effect. It means that further, well-designed trials are needed to prove its effect. A Delphi project has been completed in the UK to reach a consensus on which physiotherapy technique(s) should be considered as 'standard'. These will now be compared in a well-designed trial with a control intervention. It is difficult from the existing evidence to perform a sample size calculation to decide how many patients will be required in a placebo-controlled study to avoid a false negative conclusion, but it is likely that 300–500 patients/arm will be needed.

Occupational therapy

Occupational therapists are trained to support individuals with PD to maintain their usual level of self-care, work and leisure activity for as long as possible. Interventions may include support in re-organising the daily routine, learning new skills for alternative or adaptive ways to carry out activities, or providing and advising on specialist equipment or resources. When it is no longer possible to maintain patients' activities, occupational therapists support individuals in changing and adapting their roles. The aims of intervention are to reduce stress, minimise disability and handicap, and improve quality of life, despite the natural increase in impairment.

The Cochrane systematic review of occupational therapy in PD found that only two randomised, controlled trials had evaluated this in 84 patients. Although both trials reported positive effects of occupational therapy, major methodological criticisms (*i.e.* small numbers, inadequate placebo interventions, methods of randomisation and concealment of allocation) and the possibility of publication bias led the authors to conclude that there is insufficient evidence to support or refute the efficacy of occupational therapy in PD.

As with physiotherapy, a systematic approach to occupational therapy development in PD is underway. A Delphi project has documented how individual therapists across the UK treated patients and what techniques they felt worked best. A pilot trial of occupational therapy versus delayed therapy is underway in the West Midlands (PD OT Trial). This will inform the design of a larger definitive study.

Speech and language therapy
Dysarthria

Dysarthria is a common manifestation of PD which increases in frequency and intensity with progression of the disease. The term 'dysarthria' is a collective name for a group of speech disorders resulting from disturbances in muscular control of the speech mechanism due to damage of the central nervous system. These problems with oral communication stem from paralysis, weakness or incoordination of the speech musculature.

Common characteristics of parkinsonian dysarthria are:

- monotony of pitch and volume (dysprosody)
- reduced stress
- imprecise articulation
- variations in speed, resulting in both inappropriate silences and rushes of speech
- a breathy hoarseness to the speech (hypophonia), reflecting the difficulty the patient has in synchronising talking and breathing.

Many of these features are attributed to hypokinesia (paucity of movement).

The neural mechanisms underlying dysarthria in PD are poorly understood. Laryngeal examination by stroboscopy has shown asymmetric abductor and adductor movements and incomplete vocal cord closure in parkinsonian patients. Bowed vocal cords, which are firm rather than flaccid, have been observed during speech and may be related to the increased rigidity in the vocalis muscle and to breathy phonation. Dysynchronous vocal cord motion has also been observed and is related to hoarseness.

The speech and language therapist can treat dysarthria in PD with behavioural treatment techniques, such as drills and exercises, and with instrumental aids including prosthetic and augmentative devices.

The Cochrane reviews of speech and language therapy in PD found three randomised, controlled trials comparing speech and language therapy with placebo for speech disorders in only 63 patients with PD. However, numerical data were only available from two trials in just 41 patients. Also, changes in outcomes were not compared between the intervention and placebo groups; the authors compared baseline and final outcomes for each arm separately. Thus, in two studies the loudness of patients' voices was increased by 7–18%, depending on the speaking task being performed. It is likely that this was a clinically significant improvement. Although the degree of improvement reduced after 6 months, it was still within a clinically useful range. Other measures of dysarthria (*e.g.* monotonicity, pitch) were measured in two trials and also improved, although the clinical significance of these improvements was less clear-cut. The small numbers of patients, the methodological flaws in the trials and the possibility of publication bias prevented a conclusion from being made on the efficacy of speech and language therapists in PD. Much larger trials are required once a 'standard' approach to therapy has been agreed within the profession.

The Cochrane review comparing various types of speech and language therapy in PD found two trials in 71 patients. The types of therapy were so heterogeneous that the results could not undergo meta-analysis, but there was no conclusive evidence that one form of therapy was better than another, bearing in mind the small numbers and methodological criticisms of the studies.

> Cochrane reviews show that there is insufficient evidence to prove the efficacy of physiotherapy, occupational therapy, and speech and language therapy in PD

Dysphagia

Dysphagia occurs frequently in PD, although patients themselves may be unaware of swallowing difficulties. Several abnormalities in the various phases of swallowing have been described and include abnormal bolus formation, transfer and oesophageal dysmotility. Swallowing speed and bolus volume are significantly lower in patients when compared to age-matched controls, and decline significantly with disease severity. Dysphagia can lead to 'silent aspiration' and, although some authors have suggested that this leads to an increased risk of pneumonia which is a significant cause of mortality in patients with PD, others have found no association with dysphagia and chest infections requiring antibiotics.

Although levodopa improves swallowing speed, pharmacotherapy has only a limited amount to offer patients with more severe deficits. It has, therefore, been suggested that speech and language therapy may improve the remaining

swallowing difficulties experienced by patients with PD. Therapists provide careful assessment and diagnosis of swallowing problems. They advise on swallowing technique, provide exercises, may offer dietary alternatives, and advise on food consistency to reduce the risks of ill health and promote safety and comfort in swallowing.

> Speech and language therapy may improve the swallowing difficulties that are not alleviated by pharmacotherapy

The Cochrane review of speech and language therapy for dysphagia failed to find any trials examining this issue.

> Further trials are needed to assess the effects of interventions such as physiotherapy, occupational therapy, and speech and language therapy, and when they should be used. In the meantime, it would seem prudent to refer patients with advanced disease for assessment and treatment by a multidisciplinary team

Parkinson's Disease Nurse Specialists (PDNSs)

The concept of PDNSs has been developed in the UK by a collaboration between the Parkinson's Disease Society and the pharmaceutical industry. The first five PDNSs were introduced in the early 1990s but their success led to many other posts developing throughout the country, based both in primary and secondary care. At present, there are over 200 nurses in the UK, although the NICE guidelines suggest that this should increase to over 300.

PDNSs play a number of valuable roles:

- they provide a link between the patient and his or her carer with primary and secondary care clinicians and nurses, with allied health professionals, and with social services
- they are often in the best position to co-ordinate all aspects of the patient's 'care package'

- they are trained to be able to advise patients on their medication within the limits set by medical staff, including more complex treatment regimens such as apomorphine injections and infusions
- they can inform and educate patients, carers, other nurses and therapists, and medical staff about the condition and its treatment.

> Parkinson's Disease Nurse Specialists act as key workers to co-ordinate the patient's care package, advise on medication issues, and educate patients, carers, medical staff, and other nurses and therapists

There has been considerable debate about whether PDNSs should be based in the community or in secondary care. The precise location of their office or base probably does not matter provided their post allows them considerable access to patients in the community and access to expertise in the management of PD which is usually based in secondary care.

> Parkinson's Disease Nurse Specialists are best based in the community with strong links with specialist Parkinson's disease clinics in secondary care

The cost-effectiveness of the PDNSs has recently been evaluated in a randomised, controlled trial in the UK. In nine randomly selected health authorities, stratified by population mortality rates and social deprivation, 438 general practitioners (GPs) recruited 1869 patients with PD. Of these, 1041 patients were allocated to receive the services of a PDNS (home visits at 8-week intervals), while 818 received standard care (control group). They were followed for 2 years using blinded raters who interviewed patients in their homes to record data on quality of life and health economics.

Only one outcome measure (Likert scale of global function) showed any benefit from PDNS

intervention and this was open to bias from patients being aware of their allocation. Many other measures including those of quality of life were unchanged. This lack of improvement may have been due to: (i) nurses being evaluated too soon after their training; (ii) lack of inter-related services in the nurse's area; and (iii) low power of the trial to find small differences. However, PDNS care was at least found to be cost-neutral.

> Parkinson's Disease Nurse Specialists have been shown to be cost-neutral in a large randomised, controlled trial

The trial did find that PDNS care helped with:

- clinical monitoring and medication adjustment
- providing a point of contact for support, including home visits when appropriate
- providing information to patients and carers about PD.

The NICE PD management guidelines (chapter 13) are supportive of PDNSs. The NICE implementation package suggests expansion of the present 200 posts by around another 100 to ensure all PD patients have access to a PDNS.

Other therapies

Other therapists may be required by patients with PD at various stages. The advice of a nutritionalist (dietitian), for example, can be invaluable as unexplained weight loss and dysphagia are common in the condition. Similarly, a continence nurse may be needed for bladder disturbance in patients with advanced disease. Furthermore, a psychologist may be required to advise patients on the management of anxiety which can be a problem at any stage of the condition.

Further reading

Clarke CE, Gullaksen E, MacDonald S, Lowe F. Referral criteria for speech and language therapy assessment of dysphagia caused by idiopathic Parkinson's disease. *Acta Neurol Scand* 1998; **97**: 27–35.

Clarke CE, Zobiw R, Gullaksen E. Quality of life and care in Parkinson's disease. *Br J Clin Pract* 1995; **49**: 288–93.

Deane KHO, Whurr R, Playford ED *et al*. Speech and language therapy for dysarthria in Parkinson's disease (Cochrane Reviews). In: *The Cochrane Library*; Issue 2. Oxford: Update Software, 2000.

Deane KHO, Ellis-Hill C, Clarke CE *et al*. Occupational therapy for patients with Parkinson's disease (Cochrane Review). In: *The Cochrane Library*; Issue 3. Oxford: Update Software, 2001.

Deane KHO, Jones D, Clarke CE *et al*. Physiotherapy for patients with Parkinson's disease (Cochrane Review). In: *The Cochrane Library*; Issue 3. Oxford: Update Software, 2001.

Findley L, Peto V, Pugner K *et al*. The impact of Parkinson's disease on quality of life: results of a research survey in the UK. *Mov Disord* 2000; **15 (Suppl 3)**: 179.

Jarman B, Hurwitz B, Cook A *et al*. Effects of community based nurses specialising in Parkinson's disease on health outcome and costs. *BMJ* 2002; **324**; 1072–5.

MacMahon DG, Findley L, Holmes J, Pugner K. The true economic impact of Parkinson's disease: a research survey in the UK. *Mov Disord* 2000; **15 (Suppl 3)**: 178–9.

Parkinson's Disease Society. *Competencies: an integrated career and competency framework for nurses working in PD management*. London: Parkinson's Disease Society, 2005.

13 Management guidelines

NICE guidelines for the diagnosis and management of PD

The drive towards clinical practice becoming evidence-based has led to the production of several sets of diagnostic and management guidelines for Parkinson's disease (PD) over the last 10 years. The most recent are those produced by the National Institute for Health and Clinical Excellence (NICE) in the UK and the American Academy of Neurology. Both guidelines were developed from rigorous systematic review of the literature which was graded according to the quality of the evidence (Table 13.1). The subsequent recommendations were also graded according to the level of evidence on which they were based (Table 13.2). The conclusions of these two guidelines are similar, so only a summary of the NICE guidelines will be given here. The full version of the NICE guidelines is available from the NICE website.

Table 13.1
Categories of evidence for clinical decision making

Category	Type of evidence
1a	Evidence from systematic review of RCTs
1b	Evidence from one or more RCTs
2a	Evidence from one or more controlled but non-randomised study
2b	Evidence from one or more quasi-experimental study
3	Evidence from descriptive study(s) such as case-control study
4	Evidence from expert committee reports or opinions or clinical experience of respected authorities

Table 13.2
Strength of recommendation for clinical decision making

Strength	Recommendation
A	Directly based on category I evidence
B	Directly based on category II evidence or extrapolated recommendation from category I evidence
C	Directly based on category III evidence or extrapolated recommendation from category I or II evidence
D	Directly based on category IV evidence or extrapolated recommendation from category I, II, or III evidence

NICE guidelines for the diagnosis and management of PD

Communication

Although the evidence level is low (grade D), the NICE guidelines recognise the crucial importance of effective communication with people with PD to empower them to participate in the judgements and choices about their own care. However, discussions should be aimed at achieving a balance between the provision of honest realistic information about the condition and the promotion of optimism. Communication should be oral and written to account for potential cognitive impairment in PD. It is important that the family and carer of a patient with PD should be given information about the condition, their entitlements to care assessment and the support services available. Patients should have a comprehensive care plan agreed between the individual, their family and/or carers and specialist and secondary healthcare providers.

The NICE guidelines state that patients with suspected Parkinson's disease should be referred quickly and untreated to an expert in the differential diagnosis of the condition and should be kept under regular review by them

Diagnosis

The NICE guidelines advise that people with suspected PD should be referred quickly (within

6 weeks but with complex problems within 2 weeks) and untreated to a specialist with expertise in the differential diagnosis of the condition (grade B). They recommend that PD should be diagnosed clinically based on the UK Parkinson's Disease Society Brain Bank Criteria (Table 4.1; grade B). They also recommend that the diagnosis of PD should be reviewed regularly (6–12 monthly) and be reconsidered if atypical clinical features develop (grade D). NICE advises that ^{123}I-FP-CIT SPECT should be available to specialists with expertise in its use and interpretation, mainly for people with tremor where essential tremor cannot be clinically differentiated from parkinsonism (grade A).

> The NICE guidelines state that patients with Parkinson's disease should have access to a Parkinson's Disease Nurse Specialist

Pharmacological therapy in early PD

The NICE guidelines accept that there is no compound which has been conclusively shown to be neuroprotective in PD, but further work in this area is urgently required.

In terms of the initial symptomatic therapy for PD, the NICE guidelines state that there is no single drug of choice and that decisions need to be individually tailored to the patient after informing them of the short- and long-term benefits and drawbacks of the different drug classes (grade D). This is taken further in the algorithm given in Figure 13.1 which provides the author's overview of the drug management of PD.

NICE advises that, whilst levodopa may be used in early PD, the dose should be kept as low as possible to maintain good function in order to reduce the development of motor complications (grade A). Dopamine agonists are an alternative initial therapy (grade A), but adequate doses must be used (grade D). The NICE guidelines recommend using a non-ergot dopamine agonist or, with ergot-derived agonists, that annual monitoring of at least

renal function tests, erythrocyte sedimentation rate (ESR) and chest radiograph is performed (grade D). MAOB inhibitors are also supported by the NICE guidelines (grade A), but beta-blockers and anticholinergics for tremor and amantadine should not be used as first line therapy (grades D, B and D, respectively).

Pharmacological therapy in later PD

Since most people with PD will develop motor complications on levodopa therapy, the NICE guidelines accept the need for adjuvant therapy with dopamine agonists, an MAOB inhibitor or a COMT inhibitor (all grade A), but there is insufficient evidence on which to base a choice between these. This is taken further in the algorithm given in Figure 13.1.

Amantadine was supported by the NICE guidelines for the management of dyskinesia (grade C) and apomorphine injections (grade B) and infusions (grade D) for severe motor complications.

The NICE guidelines highlighted a number of generic issues with anti-parkinsonian medication (all grade D):

1. Treatment should not be withdrawn abruptly or allowed to fail suddenly due to poor absorption (*e.g.* gastroenteritis, abdominal surgery) to avoid acute akinesia or neuroleptic malignant syndrome.

2. Withdrawing patients from their antiparkinsonian drugs ('drug holidays') to reduce motor complications should not be undertaken because of the risk of neuroleptic malignant syndrome.

3. In view of the risks of sudden changes in antiparkinsonian medication, people with PD who are admitted to hospital or care homes should have their medication given at the appropriate times, which may mean allowing self-medication and adjusted by, or adjusted only after discussion with, a specialist in the management of PD.

4. Dopamine dysregulation syndrome occurs due to dopaminergic medication overuse

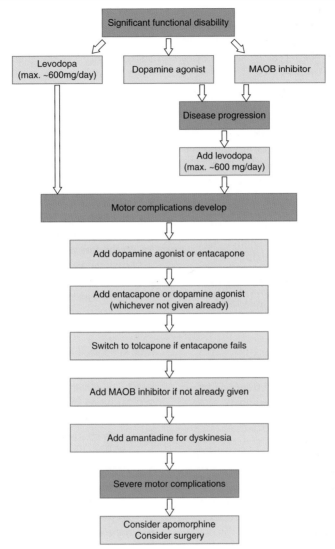

Figure 13.1
Guidelines for the drug management of PD.

leading to abnormal behaviour, including hypersexuality, pathological gambling and stereotypic motor acts.

Surgery

The NICE guidelines support bilateral subthalamic nucleus stimulation (grade D) in people with PD who:

- have motor complications that are refractory to best medical treatment
- are biologically fit with no clinically significant active co-morbidity
- are levodopa responsive
- have no clinically significant active mental health problems, for example, depression or dementia.

The NICE guidelines state that patients with Parkinson's disease should have access to physiotherapy, occupational therapy and speech and language therapy when required

Non-motor features

Mental health problems

The NICE guidelines recognise the difficulties in diagnosing depression in PD and that there is little evidence on which drug class should be used to treat it (grade D). The guidelines provide a management regimen for psychosis in PD as suggested in Table 10.1. NICE provide a cautious recommendation that 'cholinesterase inhibitors have been used successfully in individual people with PD dementia', but 'further research is recommended to identify those patients who will benefit from this treatment' (grade D).

Others

The NICE guidelines advice on managing sleep disorders, falls and autonomic dysfunction in PD is of low grade (D) and follows that suggested in chapter 10.

Allied health professionals and nursing interventions

The NICE guidelines support the provision of Parkinson's Disease Nurse Specialists (grade C) to provide:

- clinical monitoring and medication adjustment
- a continuing point of contact for support, including home visits, when appropriate
- a reliable source of information about clinical and social matters of concern to people with PD and their carers.

Support is also given to physiotherapy in PD (grade B), in particular for:

- gait re-education, improvement of balance and flexibility

- enhancement of aerobic capacity
- improvement of movement initiation
- improvement of functional independence, including mobility and activities of daily living
- provision of advice regarding safety in the home environment.

Occupational therapy in PD is supported by the NICE guidelines (grade D), in particular for:

- maintenance of work and family roles, home care and leisure activities
- improvement and maintenance of transfers and mobility
- improvement of personal self-care activities, such as eating, drinking, washing and dressing
- environmental issues to improve safety and motor function
- cognitive assessment and appropriate intervention.

NICE supported speech and language therapy in PD to:

- improve vocal loudness and pitch range, including speech therapy programmes such as Lee Silverman Voice Treatment (grade B)
- teach strategies to optimise speech intelligibility (grade D)
- ensure an effective means of communication is maintained throughout the course of the disease, including use of assistive technologies (grade D)
- review and management to support safety and efficiency of swallowing and to minimise the risk of aspiration (grade D).

Palliative care

The NICE guidelines acknowledge the palliative care requirements of people with PD which should be considered throughout all phases of the disease (grade D). Whilst this includes end-of-life issues, palliative care can be appropriate earlier in the illness (*e.g.* onset of functionally disabling dementia, onset of significant falls).

The NICE guidelines state that palliative care issues in Parkinson's disease should be considered throughout all phases of the condition

Further reading

American Academy of Neurology. Practice Parameters for Parkinson's disease. *Neurology* 2006; **66**: 968–1002.

Miyasaki JM, Martin W, Suchowersky O *et al*. Practice parameter: initiation of treatment for Parkinson's disease. *Neurology* 2002; **58**: 11–7.

National Collaborating Centre for Chronic Conditions. *Parkinson's disease – National clinical guideline for diagnosis and management in primary and secondary care*. London: Royal College of Physicians, 2006. NICE website: <http://www.nice.org>.

Useful addresses and information

Charities
Reference books
Websites

Charities

Parkinson's Disease Society of the United
Kingdom
215 Vauxhall Bridge Road, London
SW1V 1EJ, UK
Tel: +44 (0)20 7931 8080
Fax: +44 (0)20 7233 9908
E-mail: enquiries@parkinsons.org.uk
Helpline: +44 (0)808 800 0303
E-mail: branch.info@parkinsons.org.uk for
details of local officer and/or branch.

Parkinson's Disease Society, Scottish Office
Forsyth House, Lommond Court, Castle Business
Park, Stirling FK9 4TU, UK
Tel/Fax: +44 (0)1786 433811
Email: pds.scotland@parkinsons.org.uk

Parkinson's Disease Society, Wales Office
c/o Interlink Maritime Offices, Woodland
Terrace, Maesycoed, Pontypridd CF37 1DZ, UK
Tel: +44 (0)1443 404916
Email: pds.wales@parkinsons.org.uk

Parkinson's Association of Ireland
Carmichael House, North Brunswick Street,
Dublin 7, Ireland
Freephone 1 800 359 359

YAPPRS (Young Active Parkinsonians, Partners
and Relatives)
c/o Emma Bennion, Church Farm, Bircham
Newton, King's Lynn, Norfolk PE31 6QZ, UK
Tel/Fax: +44 (0)1485 578592

European Parkinson's Disease Association
Lizzie Graham, EPDA Liaison/Project Manager, 4
Golding Road, Sevenoaks, Kent TN13 3NJ, UK
Tel/Fax: +44 (0)1732 457 683
E-mail: admin@epda.eu.com

Movement Disorder Society
International Secretariat, 555 East Wells Street,
Suite 1100, Milwaukee, WI 53202-3823, USA
Tel: +1 414 276 2145
Fax: +1 414 276 3349
E-mail: info@movementdisorders.org

Reference books

Playfer J, Hindle J. (eds) *Parkinson's Disease in
the Older Patient*. London: Arnold, 2001.

Quinn NP. (ed) *Parkinsonism*. London: Baillière
Tindall, 1997.

Watts RL, Koller WC. (eds) *Movement Disorders*,
2nd edn. New York: McGraw-Hill, 2004.

Websites

www.parkinsons.org.uk

UK Parkinson's Disease Society website for
patients and staff.

www.parkinsonsdisease.com

Awakenings site of European Parkinson's
Disease Association – useful for staff and
patients.

www.parkinsonsinfo.com

Information service for patients.

www.young-parkinsons.org.uk

Information service for younger patients.

www.parkinson.org

National Parkinson Foundation – North
American Parkinson's disease society website
for patients and staff.

www.pdf.org

Parkinson's Disease Foundation – another North
American Parkinson's disease society website
for patients and staff.

www.pdmed.bham.ac.uk

PD MED trial website.

www.pdsurg.bham.ac.uk

PD SURG trial website.

Index

Page numbers in *italics* refer to information that is shown only in a table or diagram.